Introduction to Well Control

SECOND EDITION

by Daniel Diener

Published by

THE UNIVERSITY OF TEXAS
CONTINUING EDUCATION
PETROLEUM EXTENSION SERVICE
Austin, Texas

1999

Library of Congress Cataloging-in-Publication Data

Diener, Daniel, 1941–
    Introduction to well control / by Daniel Diener. — 2nd ed.
        p.   cm.
    ISBN 0-88698-185-9
    1.   I. Title.
    TN870.V28   1997   97-10098
        665.5—dc21   CIP

Catalog No. 5.10020
ISBN 0-88698-185-9

The University of Texas at Austin is an equal opportunity employer.
No state funds were used to produce this manual.

Table of Contents

Foreword

Petroleum Extension Service (PETEX) released the first edition of an *Introduction to Well Control* in 1981. Written by Dan Diener, a PETEX instructional designer, it was presented in a self-instructional format with spaces for students to fill in as they read the text. The idea was to make students think about the facts they were reading and react to them by attempting to correctly fill in blank spaces. It was a successful exercise for those who took the time to work their way through the material.

Since the first edition's release, however, new outlooks and perceptions have replaced the old in the field of well control. What is more, many students expressed the desire to have a "straight" text, instead of a self-instructional manual, covering fundamentals of well control.

Consequently, this second edition of an *Introduction to Well Control* has been updated to reflect the latest well-control principles and technology and is presented as straight text. While the second edition is largely based on the content of the first edition, it has many changes and improvements. The second edition also includes SI units as well as English units of measurement, because SI units are used practically everywhere in the world except the United States. Questions are provided as an aid to those who may wish to test their perception and retention of the material.

This book could not have been revised without the input from experienced well-control specialists from all over the world. PETEX would particularly like to thank Tom Thomas, Sedco Forex, who not only read the manuscript and checked it for technical correctness, but also provided input for many of the drawings; Aberdeen Drilling Schools and Well Control Training Centre, who checked it for technical errors; Triton Engineering staff, who also looked at it from a technical stand-point; and a reviewer who, although he or she prefers anonymity, went over the book with a fine-tooth comb and made many helpful suggestions.

Also to be commended for their excellent work are those on the PETEX staff who took a raw manuscript and made it into this book. Kathryn Roberts edited and organized the material to make it ready for Debbie Caples, PETEX's layout designer, typesetter, photo gatherer, etc. Doris Dickey did her usual amazing job at proofreading the text to ensure that virtually every typographical error was corrected before the printer got the book.

In spite of the assistance PETEX received from those mentioned above and from others in the industry too numerous to mention, PETEX remains solely responsible for the content of this book. While every effort was made to ensure correctness, errors seem ever able to creep into texts such as this one. Petroleum Extension Service will be most grateful to hear from those who detect mistakes and misleading or unclear statements.

Finally, bear in mind that this book is intended as a training aid only and nothing contained in it should be considered as approval or disapproval of any specific product or practice.

Ron Baker
Director, Petroleum Extension Service

PART I
Causes of a Kick

INTRODUCTION

A blowout rising to the surface can be a spectacular event (fig. 1). Many barrels of fluid can move up the hole and to the surface under tremendous pressure. A blowout is the uncontrolled release of formation fluids under high pressure. Before a well blows out, it kicks. A kick is the entry of enough formation fluids into the wellbore so that when the driller shuts in the well (stops the mud pumps and completely seals the well), the intruded fluids exert pressure in the well. If crew members fail to recognize that the well has kicked and do not take proper steps to control it, it can blow out.

Blowouts can destroy expensive drilling rigs, cause the loss of large amounts of oil and gas, and bring about serious injury or death to members of the drilling crew. Most petroleum fluids (hydrocarbons) ignite easily; so, if they reach the surface, a fire usually results. Not all blowouts reach the surface, however. Sometimes, formation fluids can flow into another underground formation at a different depth from the flowing formation. This kind of flow is an underground blowout and can be very difficult to control.

Most blowouts occur because somebody made a mistake. So, a drilling crew that is trained to (1) recognize the warning signs of a kick, (2) take proper steps to shut in and control the well when it kicks, (3) install blowout prevention equipment correctly, and (4) maintain the equipment so that it works correctly when needed, can prevent most blowouts. The key to preventing blowouts is recognizing and controlling kicks before they become blowouts.

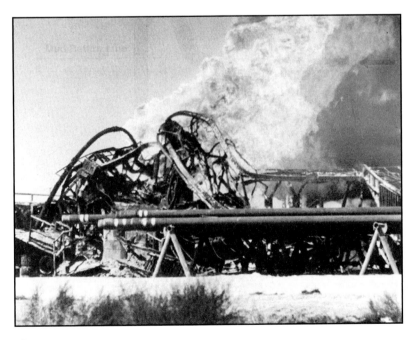

Figure 1.

1

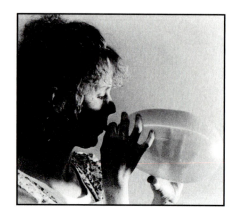

Figure 2.

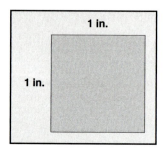

Figure 3.

PRESSURE CHARACTERISTICS

Before studying how to control a kick, let's look at a few characteristics of pressure. Pressure is the force of one object or substance against another. Blowing up a balloon (fig. 2) shows pressure at work. As air enters the balloon, the pressure inside increases and forces the elastic skin of the balloon to expand. The elastic skin resists this expansion. The balloon continues to expand until the pressure of the air and the resisting force of the balloon's skin are about equal. Reducing the amount of air causes the pressure to drop and the balloon to get smaller. On the other hand, add enough air and the pressure inside the balloon increases until the elastic skin cannot expand any farther. The balloon explodes, or bursts.

People in the United States commonly measure pressure in pounds of force exerted on 1 square inch of area. One square inch is a square that measures 1 inch on each of its sides. Figure 3 is a square that has an area of 1 square inch. Where pounds per square inch is used to measure pressure, the pressure measured is that which is exerted only on 1 square inch, regardless of the total size of the area. The abbreviation for pounds per square inch is psi.

Outside the U.S., pressure is measured in other ways. For example, SI units are used in many parts of the world. SI stands for Système International d'Unités. The SI system is based on the metric system. In SI units, pressure is measured in pascals, which is equal to 1 newton of force pressing down on 1 square metre. A newton is like a pound in the sense that it is a way to express force. Because 1 pascal is a very small unit, pressure is usually expressed in kilopascals or megapascals. (Kilo means 1 thousand and mega means 1 million. So 1 kilopascal is 1,000 pascals and 1 megapascal is 1,000,000 pascals.) The abbreviation for kilopascals is kPa; for megapascals it is MPa. A newton is abbreviated as N.

Figure 4 represents pressure being exerted on an area. At *A*, a weight of 10 pounds is pressing down (is being exerted) on 1 square inch, so 10 psi is being exerted on area *A*. Ten psi is also being exerted on area *B*. At *B*, 40 psi is being exerted on a square that is 2 inches on each side. The square thus has an area of 4 square inches, because 2 inches × 2 inches = 4 square inches. So, four times the force is being placed on *B* than that placed on *A* (40 pounds vs. 10 pounds). But *B* still has the same amount of pressure in psi—in this case, 10. The same holds true for the SI system. At *C*, a force of 10 newtons applied to 1 square metre equals 10 pascals and, at *D*, a force of 40 newtons applied to 4 square metres still equals 10 pascals because we are measuring the force on 1 square metre.

Figure 5A is a 4-inch square that is divided into sixteen 1-inch squares. To determine the amount of pressure exerted on the entire area, we measure the amount of force on only one square. Figure 5B is a 4-metre square that is divided into sixteen 1-metre squares. Just as in the English system of measurement, to determine the amount of pressure exerted on the entire area, we measure the amount of force on only one square.

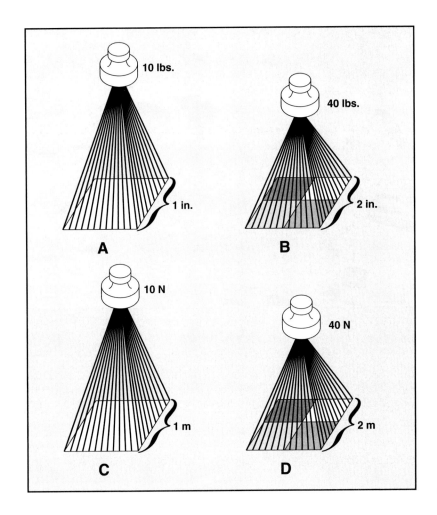

Figure 4.

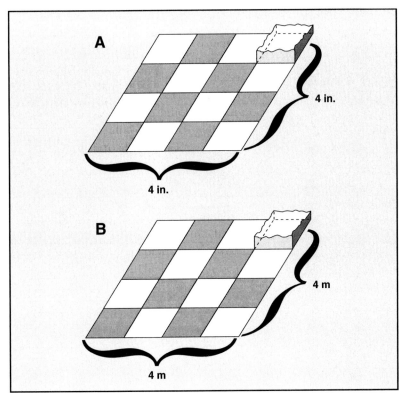

Figure 5.

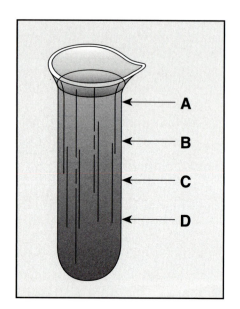

Figure 6.

Hydrostatic Pressure

The term *hydrostatic* describes the pressure a fluid exerts. A fluid is either a gas or a liquid. Hydrostatic comes from the words *hydro*, which means water or liquid, and *static*, which means at rest. So, the pressure of a fluid or liquid standing still is called hydrostatic pressure. The deeper the measurement is taken, the greater the hydrostatic pressure. For example, the container in figure 6 is full of liquid. The letter *D* is opposite the greatest hydrostatic pressure. *A* is opposite the lowest hydrostatic pressure. The amount of hydrostatic pressure a fluid exerts depends on its depth.

Figure 7 shows three containers of different shapes and sizes. All contain liquid. Container *B* has the greatest hydrostatic pressure at its bottom. The hydrostatic pressure depends on the depth of the fluid, not on the shape of the container or on total area of the fluid. A large shallow lake has less hydrostatic pressure than a deep well. Container *A* has the least hydrostatic pressure on bottom. If we measure the hydrostatic pressure in each of the containers at line *K*, the pressure in all three is the same. Remember that the amount of hydrostatic pressure depends on the depth at which it is measured. You may have experienced hydrostatic pressure when swimming in a deep pool or lake. The deeper you swim under the water, the more hydrostatic pressure you feel. Usually, you feel hydrostatic pressure on your ears.

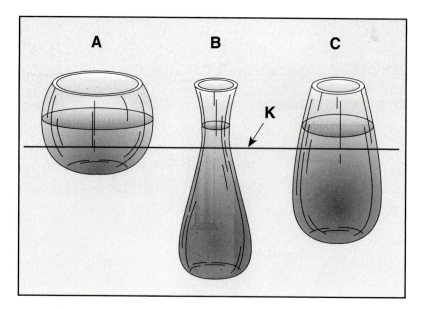

Figure 7.

Now let's see what hydrostatic pressure has to do with well control. Figure 8 shows two wells. The depth of each well is 10,000 feet (3,048 metres), and both wells are filled with the same type of drilling mud. Well *A* has 7⅝-inch (193.68-millimetre) diameter casing, and well *B* has 13⅜-inch (339.73-millimetre) diameter casing. Which well has the greater hydrostatic pressure on bottom? The answer is that the pressure in psi (or in kPa) at the bottom of well *A* is exactly the same as well *B*. Both wells are the same depth and both are full of mud that weighs the same. Therefore, the pressure at the bottom of each well is the same. The diameter of the well does not affect hydrostatic pressure.

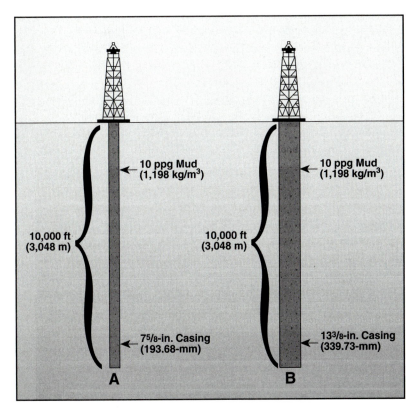

Figure 8.

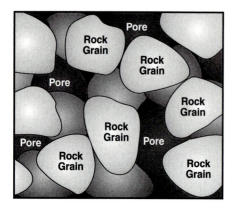

Figure 9.

Formation Pressure

Both the fluid in the formation and the drilling mud in the wellbore are under hydrostatic pressure. However, rig crews generally use different terms to distinguish between them. In a discussion of well control, formation pressure refers to the fluid pressure in the formation rock and hydrostatic pressure describes the pressure of noncirculating drilling fluid in the wellbore.

Porosity and Permeability

Formation fluids do not exist in large lakes or pools, but are squeezed into tiny pore spaces between the small grains of rock, as shown in figure 9. Porous rock, such as sandstone, can hold water or other fluids just as a sponge can hold water or other fluids. A rock with pores has porosity. Pore spaces in a rock are sometimes connected so that the fluids are able to move through the rock. Rocks with connected pores are permeable and have permeability. Porous and permeable rocks often contain fluids such as salt water, oil, and gas. Sometimes, porous and permeable rocks may have only one of the fluids or they may have two or all three.

True Vertical Depth

In formations that are permeable (have connected pores), and if the formation eventually outcrops on the surface or lies next to permeable formations that outcrop, the weight of the rock has no effect on fluid pressure. The pressure caused by the weight of overlying rocks is relieved where the formation directly or indirectly outcrops to the atmosphere on the surface. (Later, we'll discuss what can happen when a formation does not outcrop.)

In figure 10, a porous and permeable formation that has fluids in it lies under other formations and outcrops to the surface. The weight of the overlying rocks presses down on the porous and permeable formation but, since the formation eventually outcrops to the surface, the outcrop relieves the pressure caused by the weight of the overlying rocks. Just like

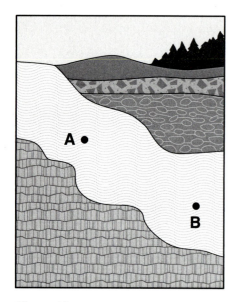

Figure 10.

fluids in a hole, the fluids in a formation still exert hydrostatic or formation pressure. Formation pressure is greater at point B than at point A. Point B is deeper than point A.

The amount of formation pressure and hydrostatic pressure depend on the true vertical depth (TVD) at which these pressures are measured. TVD is the depth along a straight vertical line from the surface to the point of measurement. Remember that vertical means perpendicular to the surface. Figure 11 shows true vertical depth as line A.

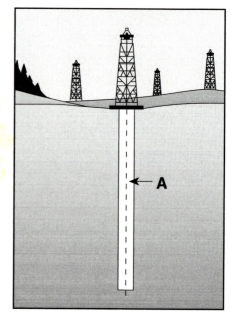

Figure 11.

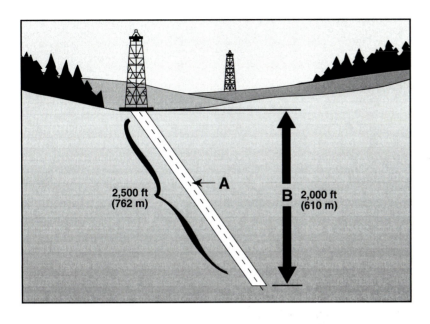

Figure 12.

Figure 12 depicts a directional well, one that is drilled on a slant and not perpendicular to the surface. Line *B* represents the well's TVD. Notice that line *B* is perpendicular to the surface and is therefore a straight vertical line—the well's true vertical depth. Line *A*, on the other hand, represents the measured depth of the well, the actual path the wellbore takes when drilled. Measured depth can be quite different from TVD. For example, in figure 12, the well's TVD is 2,000 feet (610 metres) but its measured depth is 2,500 feet (762 metres). Regardless of the well's measured depth, in well control, it is the well's TVD that is critical to pressure measurements.

How about the directional well in figure 13? Line *B* represents the true vertical depth of the well. Line *A* represents measured depth. Line *C* represents the depth of the vertical part of the well. Again, line *B*, which represents the well's TVD, is the critical depth for pressure determinations.

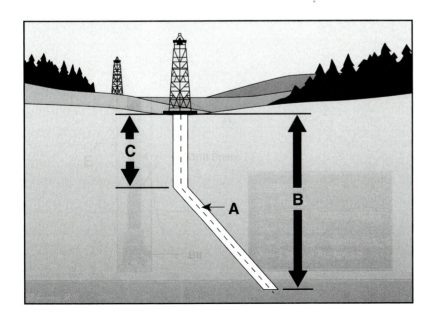

Figure 13.

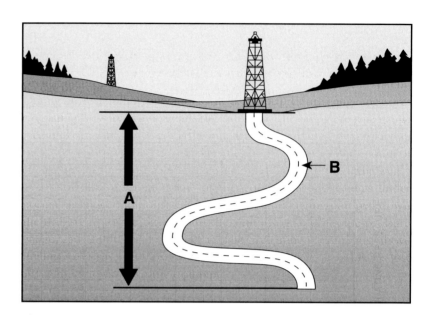

Figure 14.

The driller in figure 14 obviously had a little trouble. Line *A* represents the true vertical depth. Line *B* represents measured depth. Directional wells can be confusing. For instance, look at figure 15. Which of the two wells has the greater formation pressure? If you chose *A*, you are right. If you chose *B*, you made a mistake that could result in a kick. While well *B*'s measured depth is more than well *A*'s, pressure does not depend on the length of the drill stem or the measured depth of the well. Rather, it depends on the true vertical depth of the well.

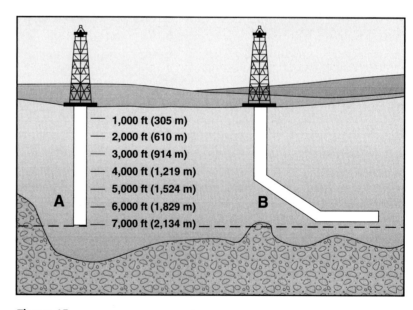

Figure 15.

Fluid Density

The true vertical depth of fluid is not the only thing that determines formation and hydrostatic pressures. The amount the fluid weighs, or its density, at a specific point of measurement also affects the pressure of the fluid. Figure 16 shows two containers. If both are full of fresh water, then the water in container *A* exerts greater pressure on the bottom of the container than the water in container *B*. Container *B* is not as tall, or deep, as container *A*. However, if we keep fresh water in beaker *A* but add enough clay and barite (a heavyweight mineral) to the fresh water in container *B*, we could increase the pressure on its bottom until it was higher than the pressure at the bottom of container *A*. So, although container *B* is shorter, or not as deep, as container *A*, we can make the fluid in container *B* exert more pressure on bottom than the taller or deeper fluid in container *A* by making the fluid in container *B* denser, or heavier, than the fluid in container *A*. Remember that the pressure of the fluid depends on its true vertical depth and on its density, or weight. These facts are fundamental to well control.

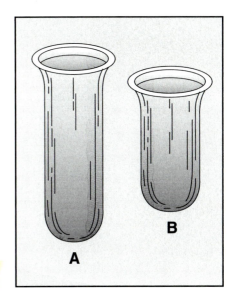

Figure 16.

Pressure Gradient

Pressure gained with depth is called pressure gradient. Pressure gradient is the uniform increase in pressure of a fluid with depth. In other words, fluid pressure for a fluid of constant density increases at a constant rate with true vertical depth. For example, if a fluid column 1 foot in height exerts a pressure of 0.4 psi, then the fluid has a pressure gradient of 0.4 psi per foot of true vertical depth (fig. 17). Therefore, for every foot of depth (from here on, when we say depth, we mean true vertical depth), the pressure of this fluid increases by 0.4 psi. So, at a depth of 10 feet, this fluid exerts a pressure of 4 psi because 10 × 0.4 = 4 psi. (In SI units, a similar pressure gradient is 9 kPa per metre of depth. So, at a 10-metre depth, the fluid exerts 90 kPa.) Now let's relate this to drilling.

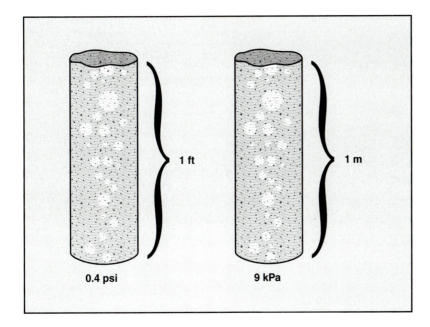

1 ft   1 m

0.4 psi   9 kPa

Figure 17.

We need a way to determine the formation pressure at whatever the true vertical depth the hole is. If we know the weight, or density, of the fluid that is in the formation (often it is salt water), we can determine the fluid's pressure gradient by consulting one of several published charts. Once we know the fluid's pressure gradient, we can calculate how much pressure the fluid in the formation exerts under normal conditions at any given true vertical depth by multiplying the pressure gradient by the true vertical depth.

For example, one type of salt water found in some formations has a pressure gradient of about 0.465 psi per foot depth. Put another way, if we measure the pressure exerted at the bottom of a 1-foot column of this salt water, it is 0.465 psi. The pressure increases by that much for each foot of depth, under normal circumstances where the formation eventually outcrops to the surface. So the normal pressure at the bottom of a formation 10 feet deep that contains this salt water is 4.65 psi; at 1,000 feet it is 465 psi and at 10,000 feet it is 4,650 psi. What is the normal pressure exerted at the bottom of a formation 2,000 feet deep that is full of this salt water? The answer is 930 psi because 0.465 psi × 2,000 feet = 930 psi. In SI units, this salt water has a pressure gradient of about 10.519 kPa per metre of depth. Thus, the normal pressure exerted at the bottom of a 1-metre column of this salt water is 10.519 kPa. The pressure increases by that much for each metre of depth, so, at 10 metres, the pressure at the bottom of a normally pressured formation containing this salt water is 105.19 kPa, at 100 metres it is 1,051.9 kPa, and at 1,000 metres it is 10,519 kPa.

Pressure Gradient and Mud Weight

In the U.S., the density of drilling mud is usually expressed in terms of how many pounds per gallon (ppg) the mud weighs. In California, however, mud density is often expressed in pounds per cubic foot, or pcf. Where SI units are used, mud weight is expressed in kilograms per cubic metre (kg/m^3). Regardless of the units used to express mud weight, mud weight affects the pressure gradient. A heavy mud has a higher pressure gradient because it weighs more than a light mud. For example, a 12-ppg (1,438-kg/m^3) mud is 2 ppg (240 kg/m^3) heavier than a 10-ppg (1,198-kg/m^3) mud. A 12-ppg mud exerts 0.624 psi per foot of depth and a 10-ppg mud exerts 0.520 psi per foot of depth. (A 1,438-kg/m^3 mud exerts 14.116 kPa per metre of depth. A 1,198-kg/m^3 mud exerts 11.762 kPa per metre of depth.) If drillers know the pressure gradient for a formation fluid, they can select a proper mud density to insure that the hydrostatic pressure remains at least as high as, if not slightly higher than, the formation pressure under normal conditions.

Let's say a well is 10,700 feet (3,261 metres) deep as it enters a normally pressured formation that contains salt water. The water has a pressure gradient of 0.465 psi/foot of depth (10.519 kPa/metre of depth); so, the bottomhole formation pressure is about 4,976 psi or 34,303 kPa (depth times the pressure gradient and rounding off to the nearest whole number). If the hole is full of an 8-ppg (959-kg/m^3) mud, which has a pressure gradient of 0.416 psi/foot (9.410 kPa/metre) of depth, this mud develops a hydrostatic pressure of about 4,451 psi (30,686 kPa) at bottom. You can see that the hydrostatic pressure is lower than the formation pressure by comparing the two pressure gradients. In this case, the formation pressure is 557 psi (3,617 kPa) more than hydrostatic pressure, so the well could kick. (A kick is the entry of formation fluids into the wellbore.) The kick could be prevented by increasing the mud weight to 9 ppg (1,078 kg/m³), which has a pressure gradient of 0.468 psi/foot (10.587 kPa/metre) of depth. The new mud weight increases the hydrostatic pressure to about 5,008 psi (34,524 kPa).

If you know a fluid's weight, you can easily determine its pressure gradient. If the fluid weight is in ppg, simply multiply the weight by 0.052. The number 0.052 is a *constant*: it is a number that does not change when used to determine a pressure gradient when the fluid weight is in ppg. The constant 0.052 is derived from the fact that 1 cubic foot contains 7.48 U.S. gallons. If a weightless cube measuring 1 foot on each side is filled with a substance weighing 1 ppg, the substance occupies 1 cubic foot or 7.48 gallons and weighs 7.48 pounds, because 7.48 gallons × 1 ppg = 7.48 pounds. To find the pressure in psi exerted on the bottom of the container, divide 7.48 pounds by 144 square inches, because 144 square inches are in 1 square foot. Since 7.48 ÷ 144 = 0.05194, or 0.052, a column of fluid that is 1 foot high and weighs 1 ppg exerts 0.052 psi on bottom.

As an example of determining the pressure gradient of a fluid whose weight is in ppg, assume that a drilling mud weighs 11.2 ppg. What is this mud's pressure gradient in psi/ft? The answer is 0.052 × 11.2 = 0.582 psi per foot.

In SI units, where the fluid weight is in kg/m³, simply multiply the weight by 0.0098. This constant, 0.0098, is derived from the fact that 1 pascal is equal to 1 newton of force applied to 1 square metre and that a weightless cube measuring 1 metre on each side contains 1 cubic metre. A newton is a measure of the gravitational force exerted by a mass. One newton exerts 9.8 kilograms of force on the bottom of the cubic metre. To find the pressure gradient in kilopascals multiply the weight of the cube in kilograms and divide by 1,000, which equals 0.0098.

As an example of determining the pressure gradient of a fluid whose weight is in kg/m³, what is the pressure gradient of a drilling mud that weighs 1,341.9 kg/m³? The answer is 0.0098 × 1,341.9 = 13.15 kPa per metre.

Another simple calculation is determining the amount of hydrostatic pressure at any given TVD. If crew members know the hole's TVD and the weight of the mud in the hole, then they can determine the hydrostatic pressure on bottom or at any depth. For example, suppose a well with a TVD of 6,872 feet is full of 12.6-ppg drilling mud. What is the hydrostatic pressure at the bottom of the hole? To find the answer, simply multiply 12.6 times 0.052; then, multiply this figure by the depth. So, 12.6 × 0.052 = 0.655 × 6,872 = 4,501 psi. Using SI units, determine the hydrostatic pressure at the bottom of a well that is full of 1,509.7-kg/m³ drilling mud and whose TVD is 2,095 metres. The answer is 1,509.7 × 0.0098 = 14.7951 × 2,095 = 30,996 kPa/m.

Well owners and drillers do not always know the pressure gradient of a formation fluid. From experience, however, they do know that most porous formations contain salt water and sometimes hydrocarbons. In areas where a lot of drilling has been going on, well owners and drillers also know the pressure gradient of the fluids that normally occur in the area.

For example, on the Gulf Coast of the U.S., drillers generally assume that normal formation fluid pressure has a pressure gradient of 0.465 psi/ft (10.519 kPa/m) of depth, which is the gradient for 10 percent salt water. In other parts of the world, this normal pressure gradient may be different, perhaps a little more or a little less than 0.465 psi/ft (10.519 kPa/m).

Here's a problem for review. Let's say we're drilling a well in the U.S. Gulf Coast and the wellbore encounters a saltwater formation at 6,175 feet (1,882 metres) TVD. If the saltwater formation is under normal pressure (we'll explain abnormal situations later), what is the formation pressure at this depth? The answer is about 2,871 psi (19,797 kPa), because 0.465 psi × 6,175 feet is about 2,871 psi (10.519 kPa × 1,882 metres is about 19,797 kPa).

Fluid Flow

Fluids under a high pressure tend to flow to areas where the pressure is lower. This fact explains why water tends to seek its own level, or move to an area where the hydrostatic pressure is equal to its own. The same thing happens underground. If the formation is permeable (its pore spaces are connected), the fluid migrates from high-pressure areas through the formation to areas of lower pressure.

Figure 18 shows two containers with the same fluid in them mounted on stands at the same height. Their tops are open to the atmosphere and a length of flexible U-shaped tubing runs between the bottom of the containers. At present, the fluid in container A is flowing through the tubing to the container labeled B, because there is more fluid in container A. But, if the fluid in B is heavier, or denser, than A, then both sides could exert the same amount of pressure and no fluid would flow between them.

What is more, by adding a weighting compound such as barite to the fluid in container B, we can increase, or raise, the fluid pressure in container B until it exceeds the pressure of the liquid in container A. If we continue to increase the density of the fluid in B, we can increase the pressure enough to cause fluid to flow from B to A.

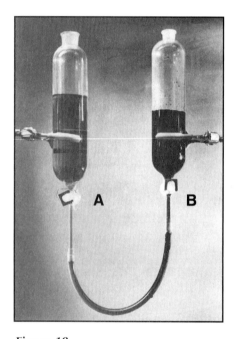

Figure 18.

CONTRIBUTING CAUSES OF KICKS

Figure 19 shows a well drilled to 10,000 feet (3,048 metres) into a normally pressured saltwater reservoir in the Gulf Coast of the U.S. At the moment, the hole is empty. It has no mud in it. The normal formation pressure at the bottom of the well is 4,650 psi (10,000 × 0.465) or 32,062 kPa (3,048 × 10.519). Nothing is in the well to keep the formation fluid from flowing into the wellbore. Crew members can prevent this kick by keeping the hole filled with drilling mud of the correct density. A hole filled with drilling mud with a density great enough to develop enough pressure equal to or slightly more than formation pressure keeps formation fluids from entering the well.

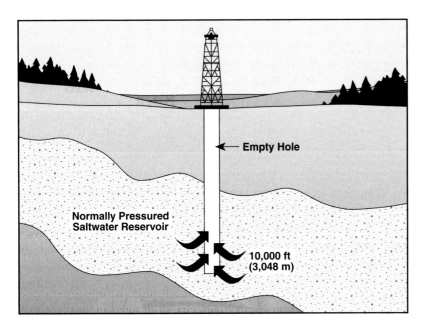

Figure 19.

Porous and Permeable Rock

A formation that contains fluids must have two characteristics before the fluids can flow into the well. First, the rock containing the fluids must be porous. Fluids are not located underground in large pools or lakes, but are found in tiny pore spaces (openings) in the rock. A nonporous rock lacks pore spaces; it therefore cannot contain fluid. Second, the pore spaces must be connected so that fluid can flow through the rock to a well. Rock formations that have connected pore spaces are permeable formations.

As mentioned earlier, nonporous rock formations cannot contain fluid. On the other hand, a porous but nonpermeable (impermeable) formation may contain fluid, but the fluid cannot flow through the rock to the well because the pores containing the fluid are not connected. In either case, a kick cannot occur. Oil companies intentionally drill into formations that are porous and permeable to locate a fluid, usually gas, oil, or both.

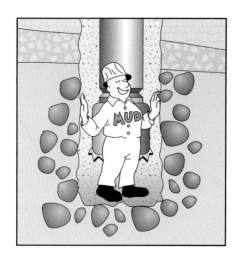

Figure 20.

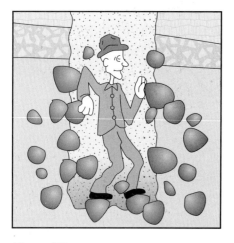

Figure 21.

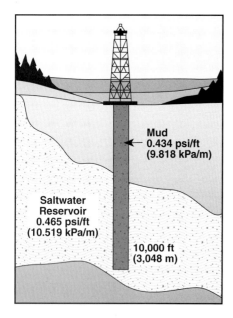

Mud
0.434 psi/ft
(9.818 kPa/m)

Saltwater
Reservoir
0.465 psi/ft
(10.519 kPa/m)

10,000 ft
(3,048 m)

Figure 22.

Drilling Mud

Drilling crew members prevent formation fluids from entering the well by keeping the hole full of drilling mud of the appropriate weight, or density, (fig. 20). If crew members fail to keep the hole full of mud, or if the weight of the mud is too low, or light, then formation fluids can enter the wellbore (fig. 21). If enough formation fluids enter the wellbore, a kick can occur. If the crew fails to take the proper steps to control the kick, a blowout can develop.

As mentioned earlier, drilling mud weight can be measured in pounds per gallon (ppg), pounds per cubic foot (pcf), kilograms per cubic metre (kg/m^3), or other units. Regardless of the unit used to measure its weight, the heavier the mud, the greater is its pressure gradient. For example, mud with a weight of 8 ppg (958.56 kg/m^3) has a pressure gradient of 0.416 psi per foot of depth (9.41 kPa per metre of depth). On the other hand, 10-ppg (1,198.2-kg/m^3) mud has a pressure gradient of 0.520 psi per foot of depth (11.763 kPa per metre of depth).

Usually, crew members keep the mud weight as low as possible—that is, they keep the mud just heavy enough to offset formation pressure. Good drilling practices require that the mud weight not be unnecessarily high. Mud that is too heavy slows the drilling rate. Mud too heavy tends to hold the cuttings made by the bit onto the bottom of the hole. Consequently, the bit redrills old cuttings instead of fresh, uncut rock and the rate of penetration drops. What is more, mud weight that is too high can break down, or fracture, a formation. In the worst case, all of the drilling mud can leak off into the fractured formation so that none of the mud returns to the surface. In other cases, perhaps only part of the mud is lost into the formation so that some of it returns to the surface. Lost circulation can be mild or severe, but it is usually not desirable to any degree.

In figure 22, a 10,000-foot (3,048-metre) well is full of mud that has a pressure gradient of 0.434 psi/ft (9.818 kPa/m), so hydrostatic pressure at the bottom of the well is 4,340 psi (0.434 × 10,000 = 4,340) or 29,925 kPa (3,048 × 9.818 = 29,925). The formation pressure at the same depth is 4,650 psi (32,062 kPa), because 0.465 × 10,000 = 4,650 (10.519 × 3,048 = 32,062). In this case, formation fluid will flow into the wellbore.

This flow is called a kick. Crew members can increase the hydrostatic pressure of the drilling mud by increasing its density, or weight. If the hydrostatic pressure of the mud is kept equal to or slightly higher than the formation pressure, a kick cannot occur. In this case, the hydrostatic pressure of the mud at the well bottom has to be about or slightly higher than 4,650 psi (32,062 kPa). As mentioned before, crew members must take care not to raise the hydrostatic pressure too much. Mud weight that is too high can slow the bit's penetration rate or, even worse, break down, or fracture, the formation. Fracturing the formation allows drilling fluid to flow into the formation and lost circulation occurs.

Keep in mind that a kick cannot take place if the hydrostatic pressure stays equal to or higher than the formation pressure. Since the depth is set, crew members have to increase or decrease the mud weight, or density, to change (increase or decrease) the hydrostatic pressure. Remember, too, that the hole must be full of mud of the proper weight. A hole that is not full of drilling mud of the right weight may not develop enough bottomhole pressure to prevent the entry of formation fluids into the wellbore. The well should be kept full of mud of the proper weight at all times.

The depth of the formation fluid in figure 23, measured vertically from the surface to the bottom of the well, is 10,000 feet (3,048 metres). It contains salt water that has a pressure gradient of 0.465 psi/ft (10.519 kPa/m). The hole has mud in it that also has a pressure gradient of 0.465 psi/ft (10.519 kPa/m). The depth of the mud measured from the bottom of the well to the top of the fluid in the well is 8,000 feet (2,438.4 metre). Since both the mud and the formation fluid have a pressure gradient of 0.465 psi/ft (10.519 kPa/m), the bottomhole formation pressure is 4,650 psi (32,062 kPa). However, the bottomhole hydrostatic pressure is 3,720 psi (25,650 kPa). This well is kicking, because formation pressure exceeds hydrostatic pressure by 930 psi (6,412 kPa).

Keeping the well completely full of mud of the proper density balances the formation pressure and prevents a kick. Anytime the mud in the hole is reduced in volume or in density, the hydrostatic pressure throughout the well decreases. If the depth of the mud column decreases, it decreases the hydrostatic pressure throughout the depth of the well.

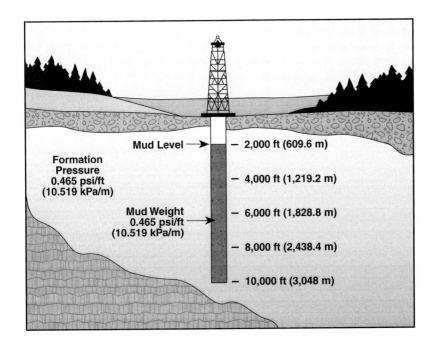

Figure 23.

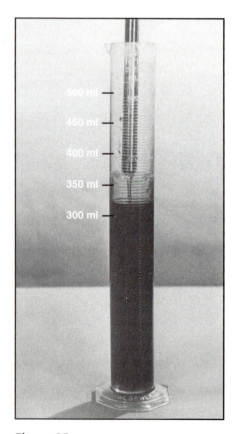

Figure 24.

Figure 25.

SPECIFIC CAUSES OF KICKS
Failure to Keep Hole Full

Drillers can make at least three mistakes that reduce hydrostatic pressure and lead to a kick. The first is simply not keeping the hole full of drilling mud when pulling the drill stem out of the hole. When the bit is on bottom, the drill stem takes up considerable space in the hole. The mud level decreases, or drops, as each stand of pipe is pulled out of the hole.

The amount of mud that should be added depends on the length of the drill stem and its diameter. On many rigs, the crew pulls drill pipe and drill collars in three-joint stands of about 90 feet (27.43 metres) each. The larger the diameter of the drill stem member, the more space it occupies in the borehole. So, 4½-inch (114.3-millimetre) drill pipe does not displace as much mud as 5-inch (127-millimetre) drill pipe. But 5-inch (127-millimetre) drill pipe does not displace as much mud as 8- or 10-inch (203.2- or 254-millimetre) drill collars. Depending on the well, rig owners may require drillers to fill the hole after three to five stands of drill pipe have been pulled. When pulling drill collars, however, good practice may dictate that drillers fill the hole after each stand.

The tall container in figure 24 holds a rod and drilling mud. The container represents the borehole and the rod represents the drill stem. With the rod submerged in the container, the mud in the container reaches to about the 375-millilitre (ml) level. When the rod is removed, the mud level decreases (fig. 25). With the rod removed, the mud level drops to about the 325 ml mark on the container. Thus, the hydrostatic pressure exerted by the mud at the bottom of the container decreases when the rod is removed. As the mud level in the container drops, so does the hydrostatic pressure exerted on bottom.

Exactly the same thing happens downhole when tripping. Pulling the drill pipe, drill collars, and other drill stem members out of the hole reduces the mud level. The drop in mud level causes a reduction in hydrostatic pressure throughout the well. If the hydrostatic pressure decreases enough, a kick could result. Therefore, the driller has to add mud to the hole to keep it filled as drill stem members (tubulars) are tripped out. The driller must know the amount of mud needed to replace the volume of the tubulars. Tables are available that show the amount of mud tubulars like drill pipe and drill collars displace. Also, many rigs have a trip tank, which is a small mud tank with an accurate gauge on it. The gauge shows the amount of mud in small divisions, such as in 10-gallon or 1-decalitre increments.

As crew members pull tubulars from the hole, the driller checks to see how much mud is needed to replace the volume displaced by the removed tubulars and adds the proper amount of mud from the trip tank. The gauge on the trip tanks shows how much mud the driller added. The amount of mud put into the hole from the trip tank should match the volume of steel pulled from the hole. It is very important to know exactly how much mud is put into the hole to replace the tubulars. The reason is that sometimes the drill stem pulls, or *swabs*, formation fluids into the hole.

Swabbing

A second common mistake is pulling tubulars out of the hole too fast. Very little room exists between the drill collars and the walls of the well (fig. 26). This space is called the annulus.

When tripping out, the driller pulls, or raises, the drill stem from the hole. When pulled up, the pipe and bit act like a piston inside a cylinder. This drill stem piston creates suction as the driller lifts it. It is similar to getting a shot at the doctor's office. The doctor plunges the needle into a vial of medicine and pulls on a plunger inside a syringe. The plunger is the piston and the syringe is the cylinder. Pulling on the plunger creates an area of low pressure where the face of the plunger piston meets the medicine in the vial. When the doctor pulls back on the plunger, it draws medicine from the vial and into the syringe. Pulling up on the drill stem too fast can do the same thing as the plunger in the syringe. An area of low pressure is created below the bit and it is possible for formation fluids to be drawn into the wellbore. This action is called swabbing.

Besides pulling the pipe too fast, another factor that contributes to swabbing is the clearance between the drill collars and the wall of the hole: the less clearance, the more likely swabbing will occur. Also, drilling in soft, sticky formations like gumbo, where the bit is likely to get balled up (jammed full of sticky clay), can also increase the chances of swabbing. A balled-up bit acts as a very efficient piston and can easily swab formation fluids into the hole.

Swabbing pulls in formation fluids. If formation fluids enter the hole, the hydrostatic pressure in the hole is reduced. If the hydrostatic pressure is reduced enough (if enough formation fluids are swabbed), the formation can kick. Formation fluids begin to occupy space in the hole that should be occupied by mud of the proper weight to control formation pressures. If the driller merely fills the hole with mud without checking whether the hole is taking the proper amount of mud, then more and more formation fluids can be swabbed. In this case, the hole is full, but it is not full of mud; rather, it is full of a mixture of mud and formation fluids. If the mixture does not develop enough hydrostatic pressure to keep formation fluids from entering the hole, the well will kick.

Since one cause of swabbing is pulling the pipe up too quickly, one way to prevent it is to pull the pipe out of the hole slowly. The best check for swabbing is to note carefully how much mud the well takes after tripping out one or two stands of pipe. Drillers should know exactly how much mud is needed to refill the hole. Checking to see if the hole has taken the right amount of mud to replace the drill stem is where a trip tank comes in handy. Drillers can check charts from tubular manufacturers to see how many gallons or decalitres the drill stem elements take up. Then, after pulling a couple of stands of pipe, they can pump mud from the trip tank into the hole to replace the pipe. The amount of mud put into the hole to replace the pipe should exactly equal the volume of pipe. If the hole takes too little mud to replace the pipe, then swabbing has probably occurred.

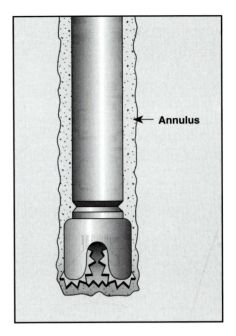

Figure 26.

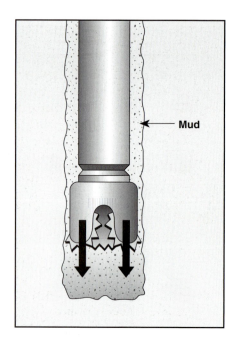

Figure 27.

Surging

The third tripping mistake drillers may make is running the drill stem and bit back into the hole too fast. If they lower the pipe too fast, surging may occur. The opposite of swabbing, surging packs the mud below the bit and creates an increase in pressure, or surge (fig. 27). The greatest pressure surge occurs immediately below the bit. Lowering the pipe slowly allows the mud to flow past the bit with a relatively small increase in pressure. If the driller lowers the pipe into the hole too quickly, the pressure surge could be large enough to break down (fracture) the formation. Drilling mud could then flow into the fractured formation, lowering the level of mud in the hole. With the mud level lowered, the hydrostatic pressure drops, and the well could kick. As previously stated, when mud goes into a formation, it is called lost circulation.

A trip tank can help drillers determine whether lost circulation is occurring when tripping back into the hole. As mentioned before, stands of pipe, drill collars, and other drill stem elements displace a given volume of mud. If the mud displaced by the drill stem as it is lowered into the hole is put into the trip tank, drillers can check the trip tank's gauge to see if the stands of pipe put back into the hole displaced the proper amount of mud. If they did not—that is, if less mud flowed into the trip tank than that displaced by the stand, it could be that mud is being lost to a formation that was fractured by surging.

Abnormal Pressure

So far this book has covered wells drilled into normal-pressure formations. A normal-pressure formation is a porous and permeable formation that contains fluids like salt water, gas, and oil and has an eventual outlet to the surface. The fluids in a normal-pressure formation exert an amount of pressure that equals the amount of pressure the fluids exert in a wellbore. For example, a 10-percent solution of salt water has a normal pressure gradient of 0.465 psi/ft (10.519 kPa/m). In the Gulf Coast of the U.S., many normally pressured formations contain such a salt water. So, in this part of the world, operators consider 0.465 psi/ft (10.519 kPa/m) as the normal pressure gradient. In other parts of the world, the normal pressure gradient may be a little higher or a little lower than 0.465 psi/ft (10.519 kPa/m).

Sometimes an abnormal-pressure zone may be drilled into, and a kick could be the result. There are two categories of abnormal formation pressures: abnormally high and abnormally low (subnormal). Subnormal pressure zones can occur in areas that have been previously drilled and completed. The producing wells in the reservoir draw down the pressure below normal. If a rig drills a new well into the reservoir (perhaps to produce, or drain, the reservoir more efficiently) the wellbore can encounter subnormal pressure. A subnormally pressured formation has fluids at a pressure that is lower than a normally pressured zone. The result can be lost circulation if the drilling mud flows into the formation. As the mud column height is reduced, the hydrostatic pressure will fall. If it gets low enough, a kick could occur.

Abnormally high-pressure zones are often located below shale formations. Shale is a type of rock formed from silt, clay, and other fine grained sediments. Shale is usually a dense rock that is porous but has very little or virtually no permeability. As layers of sediment were laid down on top of the shale, it became compressed (fig. 28). This increase in weight over millions of years squeezed the layers of shale making the pore spaces smaller and smaller and moved any fluids out of the shale, even though the shale may have had very little permeability. If a permeable formation lay adjacent to the shale, then the fluids were forced into the adjacent rock. If the adjacent permeable formation did not eventually outcrop on the surface, or was not in contact with another permeable formation that outcropped to the surface, where the buildup in pressure could be relieved, the great weight applied from above caused the fluid pressure in the formation to become abnormally high.

Thus, abnormally high-pressure formations often occur directly below shale formations. For the pressure to be abnormally high, it must be cut off from any adjacent normal-pressure formation by a layer of impermeable rock called a cap rock (fig. 29). If a rig crew unexpectedly drills into an abnormally high-pressure zone, the formation fluid would probably flow into the wellbore. This influx of formation fluids into the wellbore is, of course, a kick. Although kicks caused by abnormally pressured formations are relatively rare, they can occur unexpectedly if the warning signs that the bit is about to enter an abnormally pressured formation go unheeded.

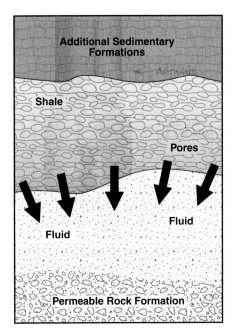

Figure 28.

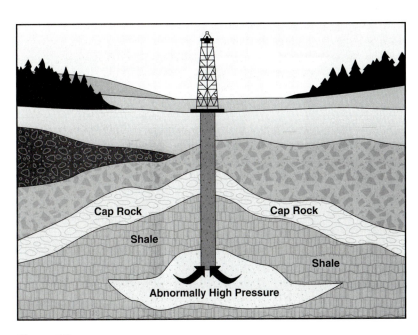

Figure 29.

S o far we have covered what causes a kick. Now let's apply this knowl-edge to the work on the rig. The main concerns on the job are discovering that a kick has occurred and then controlling it. Remember that most kicks occur in normal-pressure formations and that they are often caused by human error. Even if a kick does occur, it doesn't have to automatically result in a blowout. The key is early detection. Recognizing that a kick has occurred as early as possible lessens the danger and provides plenty of time to control it.

Kicks don't just occur. They develop in a predictable sequence of events and give several visible warning signs. This section concentrates on the warning signs you should be able to recognize on the rig floor and around the mud system.

Kicks occur below the earth's surface. You cannot see them directly, but they give clues you can see on the rig floor and in the returning mud. It is much like being on a submarine, cut off from what's happening, but having instruments, gauges, and other indicators available for guidance.

The rig's circulating system is vital to recognizing and controlling a kick. Figure 30 is a schematic of a simple circulating system. The mud pump (most rigs have more than one) picks up drilling mud from the tanks and pumps it down the drill stem and to the bit. At the bit,

Part II
Recognizing a Kick

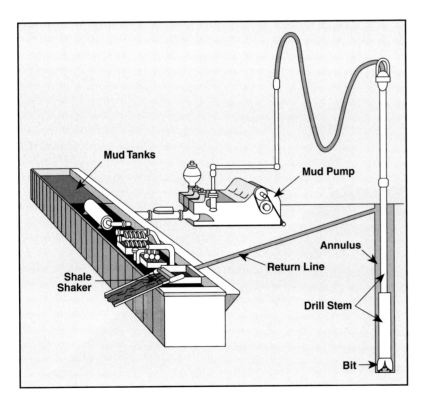

Figure 30.

the mud jets out and lifts cuttings up the annulus. The mud and cuttings go through the return line to the shale shaker, where the shaker removes cuttings from the mud. The mud then falls into the tanks and the process starts over. The mud pump must produce enough pressure to force drilling fluid through the drill stem, bit nozzles, and up the annulus to the surface.

Circulating pressure is the force that moves the mud through the system. Remember that hydrostatic pressure stands for fluid at rest. Friction does not affect hydrostatic pressure since the fluid is not moving. Hydrostatic pressure is determined by the depth and the density or weight of the fluid. Circulating pressure is determined by the amount of friction the fluid encounters as it moves through the well.

The mud pump must generate enough force to move mud down the drill stem, through the nozzles, and back up the annulus to the surface. As the fluid moves through this route, it encounters friction as it rubs against the walls of the drill stem, pushes through the nozzles, and rubs against the walls of the annulus. A considerable amount of friction is generated as mud goes through the bit nozzles. The force of the mud passing through these small openings washes cuttings away from the bottom of the hole. This action greatly increases the drilling efficiency of the bit.

In figure 31, mud enters the drill stem at a pressure of 2,000 psi (13,790 kPa). By the time it reaches the surface again, all of the pressure has been used. It leaves the annulus at a pressure of 0 psi (0 kPa). So the amount of force needed to move the mud through the well in this example is 2,000 psi (13,790 kPa). By the time the mud gets back to the surface all the pressure it began with is lost, or used up. This pressure loss usually changes with the drilling rate, mud weight, formation, pump speed, and other drilling conditions. Pressure loss does not occur evenly throughout the well. Most of the pressure is lost through the bit nozzles.

In figure 32, circulating pressure at the pump begins at 2,000 psi (13,790 kPa). By the time the mud passes through the surface piping (standpipe and rotary hose, for example) and down the drill stem, it loses 600 psi (4,137 kPa) to friction. It then exits the bit nozzles where 1,300 psi (8,964 kPa) is lost cleaning the bit and bottom of the hole. The final 100 psi (689.5 kPa) is used up as the mud flows up the annulus to the surface.

It is this last 100 psi (689.5 kPa) that concerns us most in well control. Remember that while circulating, total bottomhole pressure is hydrostatic pressure plus this pressure loss in the annulus. Suppose a 10,000-foot (3,048-metre) well is filled with 10-ppg (1,198.2 kg/m^3) mud, which has a pressure gradient of 0.520 psi per foot (11.763 kPa/m). The hydrostatic pressure at the bottom of the well is 5,200 psi or 35,854 kPa (pressure gradient times depth). But, because of the extra 100 psi (689.5 kPa) of circulating pressure lost in the annulus, total bottomhole pressure is 5,300 psi (36,544 kPa) when circulating. If, however, the mud pump is turned off (shut down), the extra 100 psi (689.5 kPa) is eliminated, and the bottomhole pressure falls to 5,200 psi (35,854 kPa). In this situation, shutting off the mud pump caused the bottomhole pressure to drop to 5,200 psi (35,854 kPa).

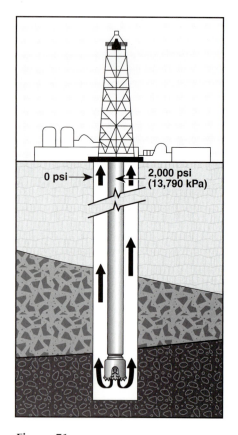

0 psi →   2,000 psi (13,790 kPa)

Figure 31.

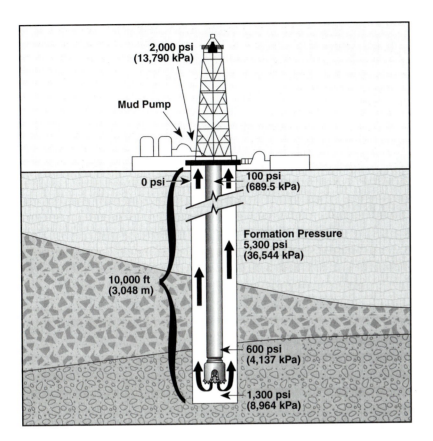

Figure 32.

If the formation at the bit is permeable and contains fluids, it is possible that this drop of 100 psi (689.5 kPa) could lead to a kick, because formation pressure is 5,300 psi (36,544 kPa). With the additional 100 psi (689.5 kPa) added to bottomhole pressure by the pressure loss in the annulus, the formation is balanced. Shutting down the pump, however, means that the 100 psi (689.5 kPa) annular pressure loss goes away, since mud is no longer being circulated. With this reduction, the formation could kick. The hydrostatic pressure must always be equal to or above the formation pressure to prevent a kick.

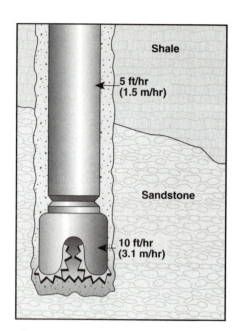

Figure 33.

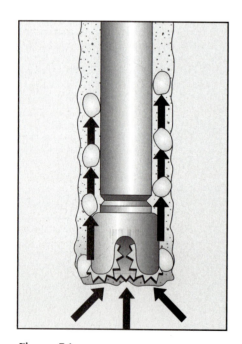

Figure 34.

WARNINGS THAT A KICK COULD OCCUR WHILE DRILLING

As mentioned before, kicks don't just happen: they occur as a predictable sequence of events. Observing one indication does not necessarily mean anything is wrong. But, if several signs are observed, chances are a kick is about to happen or one is already in the well. Knowing the sequence of events to look for is important. If one sign occurs, look for other indications. Remember that the more signals that are present, the greater is the probability of a kick.

This manual divides kick warning signs into those that indicate that a kick could occur while drilling, those that indicate that a kick has occurred while drilling, and those that indicate a kick while tripping pipe. The warning signs that a kick could occur while drilling include a change in drilling rate, an increase in rotary torque, a change in cutting size and volume, gas-cut mud, and a change in mud characteristics. Keep in mind that other kick warning signs may also occur; this book, however, covers the more obvious ones.

Change in Drilling Rate

Kicks normally occur in formations that are porous and permeable. The first indication that the bit has entered such a formation can be a change in the drilling rate, or rate of penetration. Usually, when the bit enters an abnormally high-pressure formation, the rate of penetration increases. On the other hand, when the rig is drilling with oil mud and a diamond bit, the rate of penetration may decrease when the bit enters an abnormally pressured zone. A sudden increase in the drilling rate is a drilling break. A sudden decrease in the drilling rate is a reverse drilling break.

Either kind of drilling break is a change in the rate of penetration: the depth the bit drills per hour or the number of minutes the bit takes to drill a foot or a metre. In figure 33, the bit was drilling through dense shale at a steady rate of 5 feet (1.5 metres) per hour. The bit then encountered the sandstone. Since sandstone is usually porous and permeable, it often contains fluids. As the bit entered the sandstone, the drilling rate increased to 10 feet (3.1 metres) per hour. In this case, the chances are good that the sandstone is overpressured (contains fluids under abnormally high pressure). It lies under dense shale and it is not directly or indirectly connected to the surface. A change in the penetration rate does not automatically indicate that a kick will occur, but it does indicate that a kick could happen.

A change in the rate of penetration may be slight and hard to notice, or it may be as much as a 200 percent change. And a drilling rate change may occur because the bit simply encounters a harder or a softer rock. For example, if the new formation consists of a hard rock such as granite, the drilling rate may decrease. But, as the bit enters a new formation, some type of drilling rate change will occur. A substantial drilling break suggests an abnormally high-pressure formation or that a kick has already started up the hole.

The break occurs because, once the formation pressure exceeds the bottomhole pressure, the cutting efficiency of the bit greatly increases. The higher formation pressure helps to clear the cuttings away from the bottom of the hole and pushes them up the annulus (fig. 34). Therefore, the bit is cutting into new rock with every rotation of the drill stem.

So, a drilling break is a change in the rate of penetration. It indicates that the bit has entered a different formation, which may or may not result in a kick. A radical increase in the drilling rate might indicate that a kick has already entered the well.

Increase in Rotary Torque

Rotary torque is the force needed to turn the drill stem. Most modern rigs have a rotary torque indicator near the driller's position, which shows the amount of torque on the drill stem. Torque increases with depth in normally pressured formations, but, when the bit enters a *transition zone*, an area where formation pressure is increasing above normal, rotary torque may increase. That is, more turning force is required to keep the bit and drill stem rotating at the desired revolutions per minute (rpm). In a transition zone, large amounts of shale cuttings can enter the wellbore and impede drill stem rotation (fig. 35). At the same time, the bit takes larger bites into the formation as it turns. Consequently, cuttings pile up around the bit and drill collars and cause an increase in torque. Thus, an increase in rotary torque can be a good indicator of increasing formation pressure and a potential well kick.

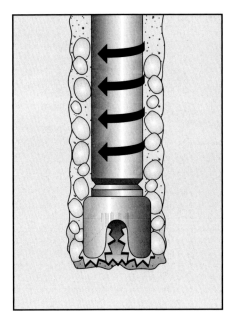

Figure 35.

Change in Cutting Size and Amount

When the bit penetrates a formation that contains higher than normal pressure, the size of the cuttings may increase. In some overpressured formations, the higher pressure in the formation causes large chunks of cuttings to enter the wellbore. In other overpressured formations, especially where the formation is made up of soft coastal or marine sediments, the cuttings may decrease in size or disappear altogether. In still other cases, the shale shaker screens may become completely covered with long slivers of shale—in oilfield parlance, the shaker becomes blinded.

Regardless of whether the cuttings increase in size, decrease in size, disappear, or blind the shaker, the important thing is that a change in the character and size of the cuttings on the shaker has occurred. The change could be a sign that the bit is about to or has entered an overpressured formation. Also, an increase in the amount, or volume, of cuttings may occur when the bit enters a formation of increasing pressure. Since hydrostatic pressure is less than formation pressure, the higher formation pressure allows the bit to drill more cuttings. Also, the higher pressure can force cuttings into the wellbore and enlarge the hole (fig. 36).

The first group of warning signs reflects a sequence of events. As a bit enters a new formation, or as a reduction in hydrostatic pressure occurs, a drilling break will often happen. If the formation is porous, permeable, and under abnormally high pressure, the drilling rate will likely increase and a kick is possible. As the drilling rate increases, it causes an increase in the number and size of the cuttings moving up the annulus. The drill stem encounters additional friction as the annulus becomes crowded with cuttings. The added friction causes an increase in rotary torque. Any difference in the shape, size, or number of cuttings will become visible at the shale shaker. It is important for crew members to immediately report any change in the cuttings to the driller. Cutting changes do not always indicate that a kick is about to occur or has occurred, but they do indicate a change in downhole conditions and that a kick may be possible.

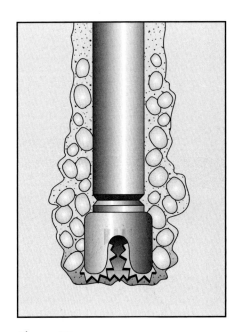

Figure 36.

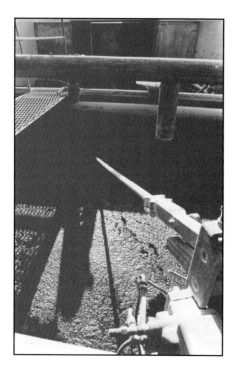

Figure 37.

Gas-Cut Mud

Another warning of a potential kick is the appearance of gas bubbles mixed with the mud at the return line or in the mud pits (fig. 37). Called gas-cut mud, this condition occurs when gas enters the annulus downhole. The presence of gas-cut mud usually means that the bit has penetrated a formation that contains gas. It doesn't automatically mean a kick has or will occur. Gas expands tremendously as it rises to the surface because the hydrostatic pressure on the gas is reduced as it nears the surface. So, what can appear as a large volume of gas in the mud tanks may only be a very small amount at the bottom of the well.

Fortunately, small amounts of gas do not affect the hydrostatic pressure enough to cause a kick. The presence of gas-cut mud does mean that the formation contains gas and has the potential to kick. So, watch carefully for any other signs.

Crew members have to treat gas-cut mud before the mud pump circulates it back down the hole; otherwise, gas is carried back down the well, and the hydrostatic pressure can be reduced to a point where a kick can occur. So that the gas will not return down the well, the mud flows through a unit called a degasser (fig. 38), which is usually located on or near a mud tank. The degasser separates gas from the mud, which can then be safely recirculated down the hole.

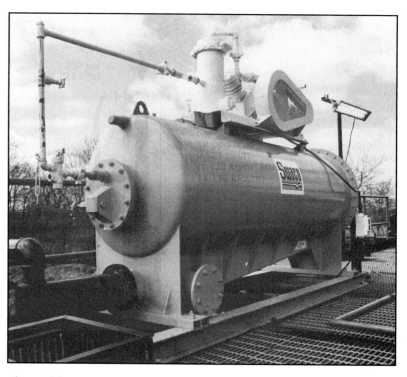

Figure 38.

Connection and Trip Gas

When the driller raises the kelly or top drive to add a joint of pipe to the drill stem (when a connection is made), swabbing can occur. Also, when the pumps are shut down to make a connection or a trip, bottomhole pressure decreases by the amount of circulating friction pressure in the annulus (annular pressure loss). Swabbing and the loss of annular friction pressure can cause bottomhole pressure to fall below formation pressure and formation fluids (including gas) can feed into the hole. A special gas detector can be installed to sense and alert the driller to connection gas. Like the entry of gas while making a connection, an influx of gas into the wellbore during a trip can occur because of swabbing or lack of annular pressure loss.

Change in Mud Characteristics

Other indications of a potential kick also occur in the drilling mud. Any change in the characteristics of the returning mud suggests that a change has occurred downhole. So, the mud should be tested periodically to find out if anything has happened. For instance, the mud engineer often performs a salinity, or chloride, test on the returning mud to measure its salt content. Increased chloride may mean that the bit has encountered a formation that contains salt water, which could also indicate that formation pressure is increasing.

Any changes in the flow properties of the mud may indicate that the hole has entered a high-pressure zone. For example, when formation pressure increases faster than the hydrostatic pressure of the mud column, more cuttings and cavings can dissolve in the mud and increase its viscosity (thickness). Also, any shows of gas, oil, or salt water in the mud indicate a change in bottomhole conditions. If crew members notice anything unusual in the mud, they should report it to the driller at once.

Before going on to the next group of warning signs, let's review for a minute. A kick occurs when formation fluids enter the wellbore. Most kicks happen in normally pressured formations. The basic technique for preventing a kick is to keep the hydrostatic pressure of the drilling mud slightly higher than the formation pressure. The mud pump provides the force to move the mud down the drill stem, through the bit nozzles, and back up the annulus to the surface.

WARNINGS THAT A KICK HAS OCCURRED

The warning signs discussed earlier in this chapter indicate the nature of conditions downhole that could lead to a kick. This section discusses signs that warn that a kick has already occurred and formation fluids have entered the well. Once a kick occurs, it is important to take immediate and proper steps to shut in the well and control the kick. Otherwise, more formation fluids could enter the wellbore and the well could blow out. Anytime drillers suspect a kick has occurred, they should immediately conduct a flow test. In most cases, a flow test proves whether a kick is in the hole.

Except in unusual operations, the pumps move drilling fluid down the drill stem, out the bit, up the annulus, out the mud return line, and into the mud pits. A flow test consists of shutting down the mud pumps, thereby stopping normal circulation of drilling fluid. After waiting a few minutes to allow the pump to come to a complete stop, no drilling mud should flow out of the well. If, however, the well has kicked, drilling mud will flow out of the annulus even though the mud pump is off. Because the kick has overcome the hydrostatic pressure of the mud, it moves into the annulus and forces drilling mud out. More time will be spent on this test later; for now, remember that it is a good indicator to determine if the well has kicked.

It is too expensive and inefficient to periodically suspend normal drilling operations and conduct a flow test. A flow test can, however, be made at each connection and only take a few extra seconds. But, there are several kick warnings that may appear during normal drilling or tripping operations. If one or more of these warnings occur, the mud pump should be shut down and a flow test conducted immediately. Now let's examine these warnings.

Increase in Flow Rate

Figure 39 is a schematic of a simple rig circulating system. During normal drilling operations, the mud circulates through this closed system. Therefore, the amount and rate of fluid flowing out of the well should equal the amount and rate of mud being pumped into the well. Of course, this is true only if the crew makes sure the well is kept full of mud. If the well is operating under normal conditions, the amount of mud flowing out of the flow line should equal the amount pumped into the well by the mud pump.

The system operates like a U-tube (fig. 40). After filling the tube with mud, suppose we pumped one more gallon (cubic metre) into side A. One gallon (cubic metre) of mud will then flow out of side B. In addition, it flows out at the same rate that mud is being pumped into side A. A U-tube operates as a closed system, as does a well under normal drilling conditions.

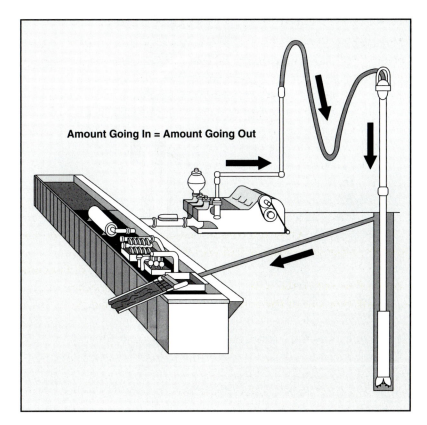

Amount Going In = Amount Going Out

Figure 39.

If a kick occurs, it forces an increase in the rate of mud flowing out of the well. Therefore, one piece of equipment many rigs have is an instrument that measures the flow rate of the mud going into the well, measures the rate coming out, and compares the two. The instrument records any difference in the rate of mud flowing out of the return line. One type of flow rate instrument is connected to a paddle and sensor in the mud return line. The paddle moves as the mud in the return line flows past it. If the rate of flow changes, the paddle senses the change and sends a signal to a readout device near the driller's position. Often, an automatic alarm system is also incorporated, which sounds an alarm when the rate changes.

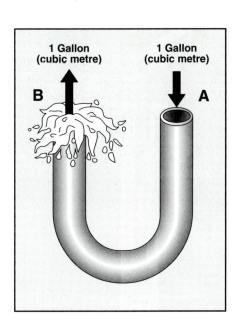

1 Gallon (cubic metre)   1 Gallon (cubic metre)

B   A

Figure 40.

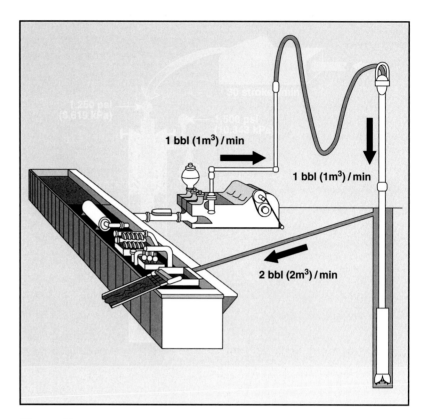

Figure 41.

Now, let's see how a kick affects a simple circulating system. Figure 41 shows the pump moving mud through the system at a rate of 1 barrel (1 cubic metre) of mud per minute. Normally, mud also comes out of the mud return line at one barrel (1 cubic metre) per minute. But in figure 41 mud is returning out of the annulus at 2 barrels (2 cubic metres) per minute. This extra fluid must be coming from somewhere.

If no one has added mud to the system, most likely fluid is entering the well from the formation; a kick is happening. If a mud flow rate instrument is installed on the rig, the increase in the amount and the rate of fluid flowing out of the mud return line is sensed by an increase in paddle movement, which registers on the readout and sets off the alarm. If the alarm goes off, the driller should shut down the mud pumps and conduct a flow test.

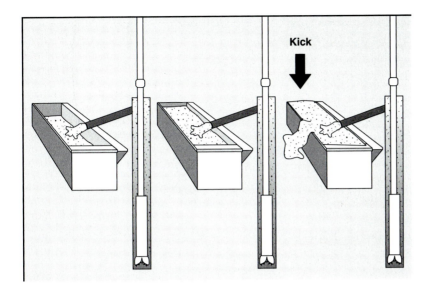

Kick

Figure 42.

Increase in Mud Tank Volume

The mud pump draws fluid from the mud tanks and forces it down the well. If a kick has not occurred, or if someone has not added mud to the system, the same amount of fluid flows up the annulus and out the mud return line. After passing through the shale shaker, the returning mud flows back into the mud tanks. The volume of mud returning to the tanks should equal the volume of fluid drawn out of the mud tanks by the pump. If a kick occurs, it adds formation fluids to the returning mud in the annulus. The result is an increase in the volume of fluid flowing out of the well and into the mud tanks (fig. 42). So, the volume of fluid entering the tanks during a kick is more than the amount drawn out of the pits. The result is an increase in the level of the fluid in the tanks.

Many rigs have a tank volume, or tank level, indicator (often called pit volume or pit level indicators, after the old-fashioned name for mud tanks, which is mud pits). With the mud tanks holding the normal volume of mud, the driller zeros the instrument to show that mud volume is neither above nor below a normal level (fig. 43). Most pit volume instruments have floats in the tanks, which send an integrated signal to a readout on the driller's console. As with the mud return indicator, an alarm may be incorporated into the system to automatically warn of a significant increase in the tank level. Any time the tank level increases, and the driller knows that it is not because someone has added mud to the tanks, the driller should shut down the pumps and make a flow check. If the well flows with the pumps off, the well has likely kicked and steps must be taken to properly shut in the well and control the kick.

An increase in the level of mud in the tanks pretty much indicates that a kick has entered the well (assuming that a crew member has not added mud to the system without notifying the driller). Unfortunately, a large amount of fluid may have to enter the tanks before it is noticed, and the kick may be well underway.

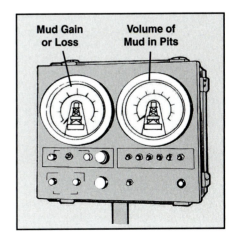

Mud Gain or Loss   Volume of Mud in Pits

Figure 43.

Decrease in Circulating Pressure and Increase in Pump Speed

Another sign of a kick is a decrease in the circulating pressure and an increase in the mud pump speed. The mud pump circulates the drilling mud, or fluid, through the circulating system. If the pump runs at a constant speed, the mud circulates at a constant speed and pressure. Usually, the driller can measure pump pressure and speed from gauges mounted near the console on the rig floor.

Once a gas kick occurs, the annulus begins to fill with a gas-mud mixture. Since the gas is lighter than the mud, it tends to help lift the mud to the surface. As more gas enters the annulus, it displaces more drilling fluid and the mixture in the annulus becomes lighter. Therefore, the mud pump does not have to work as hard to push the returning mud back up to the surface. The kick actually helps the upward movement of the fluid. These effects show up as a decrease in circulating pressure indicated on the standpipe or drill pipe (mud pump) pressure gauge and a corresponding increase in the speed of the mud pump.

The mud pump increases in speed as more gas enters the annulus and helps lift the drilling mud to the surface. When the driller or crew members notice either a decrease in circulating pressure or an increase in pump speed, and it is not because someone has changed the mud's flow properties on the surface, the driller should make a flow test immediately. A flow test can show that the well flows with the pumps off, which is a definite kick sign.

Well Flows with Pumps Off

A kick forces additional fluid up the annulus, out of the mud return line, and into the mud tanks. Shutting down the mud pump stops the normal circulation, or flow, of drilling fluid, but the kick continues to add formation fluids to the well. Remember that the amount and rate of mud pumped into the circulating system should equal the amount and rate of mud flowing out of the return line. If more mud is returning, there is probably a kick in the hole. To confirm a kick, the driller can shut down the pumps and see if mud flows out of the well without its being pumped. Shutting down the pumps to see if mud flows is a flow test. To do a flow test, the driller shuts off the pump, gives the pump a few minutes to come to a complete stop, and watches for flow at the flow (mud return) line. If drilling fluid still continues to flow out of the return line, a kick is very likely occurring.

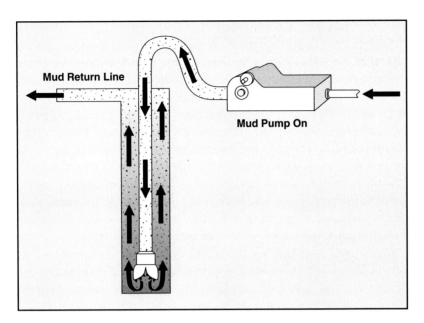

Mud Return Line

Mud Pump On

Figure 44.

Figure 44 is a schematic of normal circulation. The pump moves mud through the rig's surface piping, down the drill stem, and out of the bit. The mud then does a U-turn, moves up the annulus, and out the return line to the tanks. Figure 45 shows the pump off and the mud not flowing out of the mud return line. Just before the driller stopped the pump, the amount of mud going in was equal to the amount of mud coming out. So, when the driller shut down the pump, the well does not flow and the chances are good that the well has not kicked.

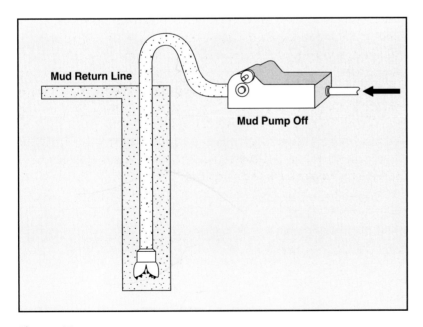

Mud Return Line

Mud Pump Off

Figure 45.

In figure 46, the mud pump is off but mud is flowing from the mud return line. A kick has occurred. The intruded kick fluids are forcing mud up the annulus and out the return line to the mud tanks. If anyone suspects that the well has kicked, the driller can confirm or deny it by shutting down the mud pump and checking for flow. If mud discharges from the mud return line, then a kick is most likely in progress. To finally confirm a kick, the driller can shut in the well completely. With the well totally sealed off (shut in) and the pumps off, the driller can then look at the standpipe gauge, which, since it is directly linked to the drill stem, indicates pressure if the well has kicked. This manual will discuss shut-in pressure in detail later. For now, just remember that if pressure appears on the standpipe gauge and the well is completely shut in, then an influx of formation fluids (a kick) has occurred.

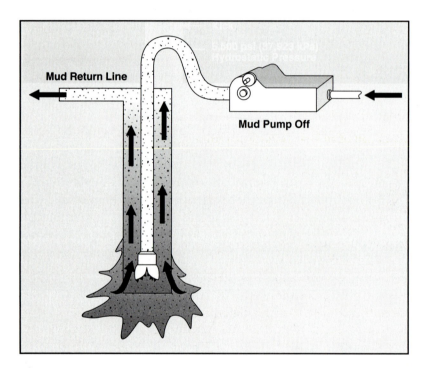

Figure 46.

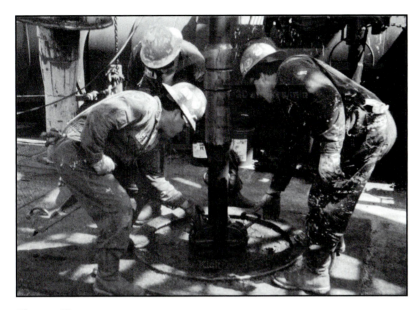

Figure 47.

WARNINGS WHEN TRIPPING

About half of all kicks occur when tripping pipe (fig. 47). The crew has a harder time detecting kicks at this time because the mud pump is usually off and there is no circulation of drilling fluid. In addition, the mud level in the well increases and decreases as pipe is tripped in or out. If a kick does occur while tripping, it is almost always the result of human error. For some reason the hydrostatic pressure in the hole is allowed to drop, and formation fluids enter the well.

First, let's review what can cause a kick while tripping out of the hole. Three different things can affect the hydrostatic and bottomhole pressure during this operation. To begin with, the driller must shut down the mud pump, which eliminates the circulating pressure loss in the annulus. Recall that this pressure loss is usually relatively small—50 to 200 psi (345 to 1,379 kPa)—but, when the pumps are stopped, a drop, or decrease, in bottomhole pressure occurs. In some cases, this pressure decrease, although it is usually small, could reduce bottomhole pressure enough to allow a kick.

Second, pulling the stand out too quickly can cause swabbing. As you recall, swabbing is the bit and drill stem's pulling formation fluids into the wellbore as they are removed from the hole. If too much formation fluids are swabbed, the fluids reduce the drilling mud's density, and thus the hydrostatic pressure, so much that a kick can occur.

Third, as stands of pipe are removed from the hole, the mud level in the hole is reduced. The hole must be periodically refilled, or a drop in hydrostatic pressure occurs. Further, the driller must keep accurate track of how much mud is being put into the hole to replace the drill stem. The hole may be full of fluid, but it may not be all drilling mud if formation fluids have been swabbed.

The driller and crew must be aware of what causes hydrostatic pressure to drop so they can take the necessary precautions. Keep in mind that the three primary causes of a drop in hydrostatic pressure when tripping out of the hole are (1) shutting off the pump which eliminates the additional pressure of circulating pressure loss in the annulus, (2) swabbing, and (3) pulling stands of pipe, which reduces the mud level.

Hole Fails to Take Right Amount of Mud

From a well-control standpoint, one of the main concerns when tripping out is to ensure that the hole takes the correct amount of mud when it is periodically refilled (fig. 48). One indication that a kick can happen or already has happened is when the hole takes too much or too little mud. If it takes too little mud to fill the hole to replace the pipe pulled, then it is likely that formation fluids have been swabbed into the wellbore. If it takes too much mud to fill the hole to replace the pipe put in, then it is possible that lost circulation is occurring. Lost circulation lowers the level of mud in the hole and thus reduces hydrostatic pressure. The driller should know exactly how much mud needs to be pumped into the well to replace the stands of drill stem that were tripped out. Because they

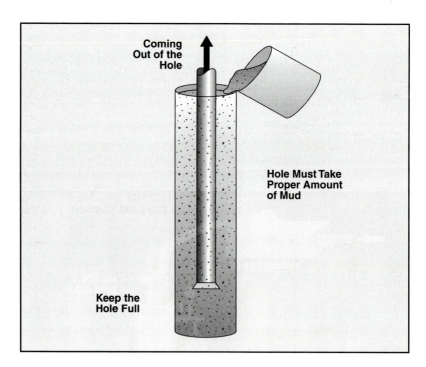

Figure 48.

are so vital to well control during trips, many contractors and operators require that the rig have a trip tank. Recall that a trip tank is a relatively small mud tank that is marked in small volume increments, such as ¼ or ½ barrel (bbl) or in decalitres (dL). When used with a trip sheet (fig. 49), a trip tank allows the driller to accurately track the amount of mud put into the hole to replace the drill stem. The trip sheet in figure 49 allows the driller to fill in the displacement of drill stem components, such as the drill collars and drill pipe; the number of stands pulled; and calculated versus actual amounts of fill-up mud.

RIG: _____   DATE: _____

WELL: _____   TIME: _____

DRILLER: _____   **TRIP SHEET**   DEPTH: _____

REASON FOR THE TRIP: _____

Number of stands to have top of DC's one DP stand below BOP's: _____

PULL ON:	✓
EVEN	
SINGLE	
DOUBLE	

DISPLACEMENT:	DC1	DC2	OTHER	HWDP	DP1	DP2
Size						
bbl/ft or						
bbl/stand						
x ft or stands						
= Vol. (bbls)						

STAND NO.	TRIP TANK GAUGE	CALCULATED Hole Fill (bbls) per Increment	MEASURED Hole Fill (bbls)		DISCREPANCY		REMARKS
			per Increm'	Accumul.	per Increm'	Accumul.	
0		███					

Courtesy of Sedco Forex

Figure 49.

In summary, remember that when the hole does not take the correct amount of mud, a kick has occurred or is about to occur. Since the level of mud in the hole falls, or decreases, as the stand is pulled out, it is very important to keep the hole full of mud. It is also important that the hole take the correct amount of mud. For every stand of pipe pulled out, the hole should take enough mud to replace the stand. If the hole overflows before the correct amount of mud is put in, then you know that formation fluid has entered the hole. Formation fluid in the hole means that a kick is about to occur or has already occurred. If the well flows with the pump off, then a kick has occurred.

Continual Flow from Mud Return Line

Tripping back into the hole presents a different situation from tripping out. As each stand is run back into the hole, it forces mud out of the return line. Once the stand is in place, the flow should stop. If the flow continues after tripping the stand in, and no one has turned on a pump or added more mud to the hole, a kick has probably occurred. Some flow should be expected when lowering a new stand into the hole, but the flow should stop for a period between stands. If mud flows continually from the well, the well has probably kicked.

This increase in flow will eventually increase the amount of mud in the pits and set off the alarm. The safety factor greatly increases if the kick is discovered earlier. It may be hard to detect the gradual increase in the pit level since some increase is expected as each stand is tripped into place. The most accurate method of determining if a kick has started is to stop tripping and check for a continual flow of mud from the flow line.

REVIEW

The following is a review of the warning signs of a kick.

Warnings that a kick could occur:

- A drilling break
- An increase in rotary torque
- A change in cutting size, shape, or amount
- Gas-cut mud
- A change in the mud composition

Warnings that a kick has occurred while drilling:

- An increase in the flow rate from the mud return line
- An increase in level of mud in the tanks (pits)
- A decrease in the circulation pressure
- Flow of mud with the mud pump off

Warnings that a kick has occurred while tripping:

- A hole that does not take correct amount of mud
- Mud flows between stands when tripping in
- Increase in the amount of mud in the tanks (pits)
- Continual flow of mud from the mud return line

So far this book has covered what causes kicks and how to detect them. Now it will cover what to do when a kick occurs. Obviously, crew members should remain calm and not panic. Most kicks can be safely controlled by applying known and proven techniques.

Specific procedures and equipment differ, depending on the operator and drilling company's policies, the rig's location, and the type of equipment on the rig. This part looks at general procedures and the primary methods for killing a kick. But first, let's take a closer look at what happens downhole when a kick develops.

Figure 50 is a schematic of a well. It shows some basic well-control equipment including a choke, casing pressure gauge, mud pump, drill pipe pressure gauge, and blowout preventers. It is not an exact representation of a rig, of course, but a simplified version. The diagram includes only items that directly concern well control. The mud pump is at *C*. It forces fluid into and down the drill stem. The BOPs or blowout preventers are at *E*. When blackened in future diagrams, they are closed. In figure 50, they are open. The choke is at *A*. It is closed. When open, flow is shown. When the BOPs are closed, the top of the well is shut in, and mud and kick fluids cannot be circulated through the normal route. In most cases, they are circulated out through an open choke.

The amount of force, or pressure, needed to move the mud through the drill stem and back up to the surface is called circulating pressure. This force overcomes friction as the mud flows through the drill stem, out the bit nozzles, and back up the annulus. The drill pipe pressure gauge measures the circulating pressure as the fluid enters the drill stem. In figure 50, the drill pipe pressure gauge is at *D*. During normal drilling operations,

Part III
Killing a Kick

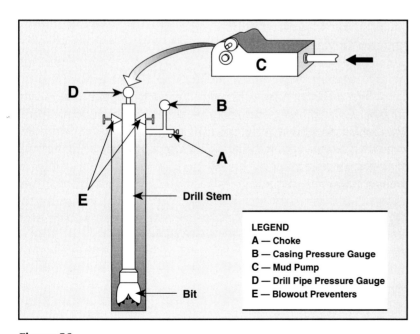

Figure 50.

LEGEND
A — Choke
B — Casing Pressure Gauge
C — Mud Pump
D — Drill Pipe Pressure Gauge
E — Blowout Preventers

Drill Stem

Bit

the casing pressure gauge measures the circulating pressure of the mud as it leaves the annulus. In figure 50, the casing pressure gauge is at *B*. Under normal conditions, the casing gauge will register zero since all the circulating pressure is used moving the drilling mud through the system. During normal drilling operations, the drill pipe pressure gauge measures circulating pressure as mud enters the drill stem. The casing pressure gauge measures circulating pressure as the mud leaves the annulus. By subtracting the casing pressure from the drill pipe pressure, we can find the amount of circulating pressure lost to friction as the mud moves through the well.

Now, let's examine some of this equipment and gauges under normal drilling conditions. Figure 51 shows mud being pumped down the drill stem, to the bit, and up the annulus. The drill pipe pressure gauge reads 2,000 psi (13,790 kPa). The circulating pressure just above the bit nozzles is 1,400 psi (9,653 kPa). So, 600 psi (4,137 kPa) is lost as the mud flows down the drill pipe.

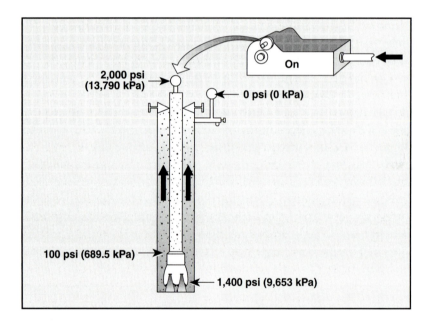

Figure 51.

After the drilling fluid passes through the bit nozzles, the pressure drops to 100 psi (689.5 kPa). Nozzles are small holes in the bit where the mud is forced through (fig. 52). The nozzles cause the mud's speed, or velocity, to increase dramatically. The great velocity helps the mud clean the cuttings out of the bottom of the hole and enables the bit to cut more efficiently. Bit nozzles work something like a garden hose. The water inside the hose is under fairly high pressure. This pressure pushes the water through a restriction, the nozzle. As the water passes through the nozzle, it increases in velocity, or speed, but loses most of the pressure. The same thing happens at the bit. In figure 51, 1,300 psi (8,963.5 kPa) is lost as the mud passes through the bit nozzles. The casing pressure gauge reads 0 psi (0 kPa). Therefore, the circulating pressure lost in the annulus is 100 psi (689.5 kPa). If the mud pump is shut off, the circulating pressure throughout the well stops, and both the drill pipe pressure gauge and the casing pressure gauge read zero.

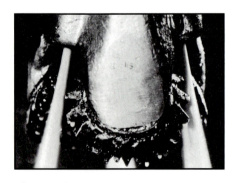

Figure 52.

INTRODUCTION TO WELL CONTROL

AN UNCONTROLLED KICK

What happens if the well kicks and the driller fails to take action? The answer is that a blowout can occur and it can occur quickly. Almost all kicks have gas associated with them. In fact, most companies tell their employees to assume that all kicks are gas kicks and act accordingly. So, what follows concentrates on a gas kick because most kicks are gas. Gas is compressible, which means a lot of it can be confined in a small area under high pressure, as in an underground formation. As the gas rises to the surface during a kick, hydrostatic pressure on it is reduced. Therefore, its volume increases tremendously, especially near the surface. As the gas expands, it moves more and more drilling mud out of the annulus, which further reduces hydrostatic pressure on bottom. As bottomhole pressure is reduced, more kick fluids enter the well. A blowout is very likely to occur if the blowout preventers are not successfully closed when the kick is detected.

Figure 53 is a simple schematic of a well. The bit and drill stem are removed to simplify the diagram. The well is full of drilling fluid that does not develop enough hydrostatic pressure to overcome the formation pressure at the bottom of the well. Since formation pressure is higher than the bottomhole pressure, a gas kick has entered the well. As the kick moves up the hole, it increases in size because the pressure of the mud on top of the kick is reduced. As the kick rises up the hole, it pushes the drilling mud up and out. Consequently, the amount of flow from the mud return line increases and a gain in tank (pit) volume occurs. An increase in return flow and a gain in tank volume are warning signs that a kick has occurred.

In figure 54, the gas has reached about halfway to the surface. A gas bubble has formed as the gas works its way through the mud. The heavy arrows at the top of the well indicate that mud is still being forced out of the well. Two arrows are shown in this illustration, although the previous one had only one arrow. The additional arrow signifies that mud is being displaced by gas in the annulus at a faster rate. Some of the gas has filtered through the mud so the bottom part of the hole is filled with a mud and gas mixture.

In figure 55, the kick has almost reached the surface. The gas bubble has increased in size. There are more arrows both at the top and the bottom of the well. These extra arrows indicate that the amount and rate of mud discharging from the hole and the kick entering the hole have both increased. The kick increases in force because the hydrostatic pressure of the drilling mud decreases as more gas enters the well.

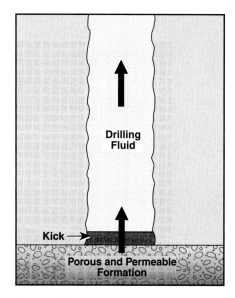

Figure 53.

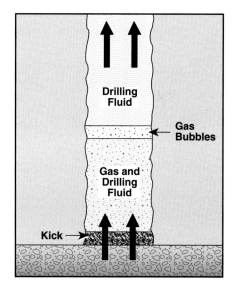

Figure 54.

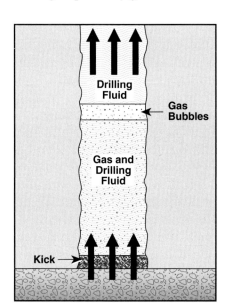

Figure 55.

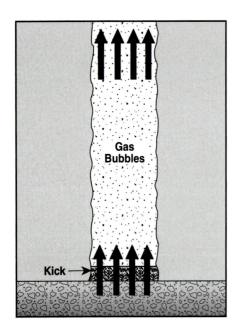

Figure 56.

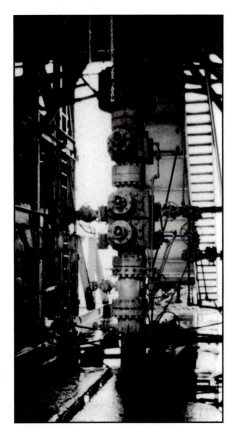

Figure 57.

In figure 56, the kick has developed into a full-scale blowout. The first step to prevent a blowout is to shut in the well as early as possible. Shutting in keeps more kick fluids (gas) from entering the well. The longer formation fluids are allowed to enter the wellbore, the higher shut-in pressure will be and the more dangerous the situation becomes. With the well completely shut in, no more kick fluids can enter the well. Circulating it out under controlled conditions can eliminate the gas that entered the well. After increasing the hydrostatic pressure by increasing the mud weight, normal operations can resume.

SHUTTING IN WHEN DRILLING

Handling a kick generally involves two stages. First, the well is shut in by closing the BOPs. Second, the kick is circulated out of the well. Shutting in the well stabilizes downhole pressure and prevents additional formation fluids from entering the well. On land rigs and on jackup and platform rigs offshore, the BOP stack is located on the surface directly above the hole (fig. 57). On floating offshore rigs, like drill ships and semisubmersibles, the stack is placed above the hole and directly on the ocean floor (fig. 58). Both surface and subsea stacks consist of several heavy-duty hydraulically operated valves. The strongest can withstand pressures of 15,000 psi. The primary purpose of the blowout preventers is to close the top of the hole.

As stated earlier, an important step in well control is shutting in the well as soon as possible. The exact steps for shutting in a well depend on the well situation and on the drilling contractor and operating company's policies and procedures. General steps can be given, however. For example, when the bit is drilling on the bottom and encounters a kick, the driller should—

1. raise the bit off the bottom,

2. shut off the mud pump, and

3. close the blowout preventers.

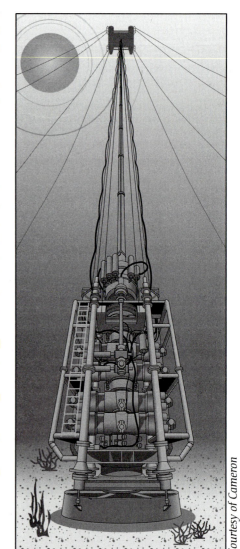

Figure 58.

INTRODUCTION TO WELL CONTROL

Other steps to take depend on the situation and policies. For instance, some companies prefer that the choke be fully opened when the blowout preventers are closed, and then closed after the BOPs close. This shut-in method is a soft shut in. Other companies prefer that the choke be fully closed when the BOPs are closed. This shut-in method is a hard shut in. Both shut in the well effectively; it is mainly a matter of preference as to which should be used.

The reason the driller should pick up the drill stem to raise the bit off bottom is to help prevent the drill stem from getting stuck and to keep the bit nozzles from plugging. When circulation is stopped, cuttings fall to the bottom of the hole. If the driller left the bit on bottom, the cuttings could pile up around the bit, perhaps plugging the nozzles and packing around the bit enough to immobilize it.

SHUTTING IN WHEN TRIPPING

If tripping pipe when a kick occurs, the situation is a little more complicated. Since the mud pump was probably off when the kick occurred, pressures in the annulus and the drill stem are the same. Therefore, the kick may flow up the drill stem, the annulus, or both. Special types of drill stem blowout preventers (fig. 59) are designed to be inserted, or stabbed, into the drill stem. Once stabbed, crew members screw the drill stem valve into the drill pipe or whatever drill stem device the valve was put into and make it up tightly. Many kinds of drill stem valves are available and they go by several names, such as upper kelly cock, lower kelly cock, full-opening safety valve, stabbing valve, inside blowout preventer (IBOP), TIW valve, Gray valve, and so forth. Regardless of their names, these preventers must be readily available on the rig floor and ready to use.

The general steps for shutting in the well when tripping are:

1. Stop tripping operations and set the slips with the tool joint just above the rotary.

2. If fluids are not flowing out of the drill stem, stab and make up the kelly or the top drive in the drill stem, and close the lower kelly cock or the built-in IBOPs in the top-drive unit. If fluids are flowing out of the drill stem, stab and make up a full-opening safety valve in the top joint of the drill stem. A full-opening safety valve enables the crew to move the valve through the fluid flowing out of the drill stem and position it over the drill stem. Since the valve is fully open, the blowing fluids can go through the valve, which usually enables the crew to stab it into the drill stem. After it is made up, crew members can close the valve to shut off flow.

3. Make up the kelly or the top drive. Once the kelly or top drive is made up, the driller can circulate mud downhole.

4. Close the regular blowout preventers.

Because the situations that occur when a well kicks during a trip can vary, the four steps are only general.

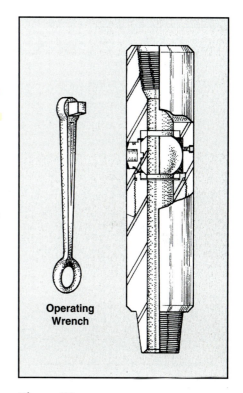

Operating Wrench

Figure 59.

Regardless of exactly how the well is shut in when a kick occurs during a trip, once the situation stabilizes, crew members can snub or strip the pipe through the BOPs to the bottom of the hole, and control of the well can be regained. Snubbing is forcing the drill stem back into the well against pressure so high that the weight of the drill stem is not enough to overcome the pressure. So, crew members use special snubbing devices (snubbing units) that apply additional force on the drill stem to get it back into the hole. Stripping is also forcing the drill stem back into the well against pressure, but the weight of the drill stem is sufficient to overcome well pressure. In stripping and snubbing operations, the driller usually forces the drill stem through a closed annular BOP. The driller allows a little fluid to leak around the annular sealing element, which lubricates the element's surface where the pipe moves against it.

CIRCULATING A KICK OUT

The second major aspect of well control is circulating the kick out of the hole by using the mud pump and the choke. The choke allows the fluid in the annulus, which usually contains the kick, to be vented while carefully controlling the downhole pressure. Many types of chokes are available, but this book covers automatic adjustable chokes.

An automatic adjustable choke consists of a special valve (the choke) that can be fully closed, fully open, or its opening adjusted to any size in between. The choke is usually installed in a series of pipes and valves called the choke manifold, which is usually some distance from the rig floor. With the BOPs closed, the driller can open a remote-controlled choke-line valve (sometimes called an HCR valve), which directs the fluids in the annulus through the choke line (pipe) to the choke manifold and automatic choke.

To operate the choke in the manifold, the choke operator does not have to be right next to the choke. Instead, the operator can adjust the choke from a remote location (usually the rig floor) by means of a choke operating device, often called a choke control panel. Adjusting the choke's size adjusts the back-pressure the choke holds on the well. By adjusting the choke, the choke operator maintains the bottomhole pressure slightly higher than the formation pressure, thus preventing additional kicks from entering the well from the formation. The mud pump provides the force to circulate the mud-kick mixture out of the annulus. So, the two primary steps in controlling a kick are shutting in the well and circulating the kick out of the hole, while maintaining constant bottomhole pressure by adjusting the choke's opening.

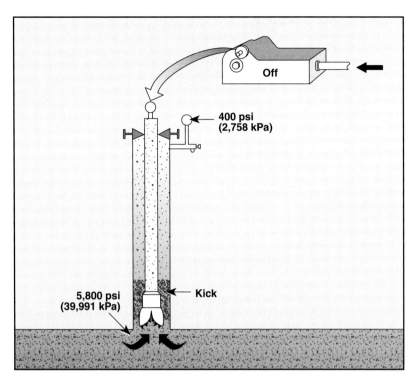

Figure 60.

SHUT-IN CONSIDERATIONS

Shutting in the well temporarily stabilizes the well—that is, completely sealing the well puts back-pressure on the well and keeps more kick fluids from entering it. It is somewhat like putting a stopper in a bottle—the pressure is still there, but the stopper (the BOPs) keep it from getting out. Shutting in keeps more kick fluids from entering the well, but the crew must gain control of the well. To see what happens if a well is shut in and no further steps are taken, look at the shut-in well in figure 60.

The formation pressure is 5,800 psi (39,991 kPa). The well is shut in (note the blowout preventers are darkened). The casing gauge reads 400 psi (2,758 kPa). Since the well is shut in, mud and gas cannot escape. But gas has entered as a kick, and it exerts pressure in the annulus. The more gas that entered, the higher is the casing pressure. With the well shut in, the pressure at the bottom of the annulus equals the formation pressure. Once this happens, the well is temporarily stabilized. At this point everyone can breathe a sigh of relief—but don't relax too much!

The casing pressure gauge registers the pressure at the top of the annulus. Under normal drilling conditions, with the well open and the mud pumps on, the drilling mud leaves the annulus at this point and the casing pressure gauge registers 0 psi (0 kPa).

The gauge in figure 60 reads 400 psi (2,758 kPa). Mud is not being circulated so there is no circulating pressure. So where does this 400 psi (2,758 kPa) come from? Since drilling mud is not compressible, the pressure from the kick transfers up the mud column and registers on the casing pressure gauge. Pressure on the casing gauge with the well shut in definitely confirms that the well has kicked.

Although the well is shut in, the gas bubble, because it is lighter (weighs less) than the mud, begins to rise up the annulus. It is similar to a helium filled balloon rising in the air. Since helium is lighter than air, it makes the balloon rise. A gas kick in the mud of an annulus is the same—gas is lighter than mud so it rises through the mud.

A gas kick rises at a particular rate, depending on the mud's properties. Let's say that it rises about 30 feet (9 metres) per minute. If the well was 10,000 feet (3,048 metres) deep, and the kick rose at 30 feet (9 metres) per minute, it would be halfway up the annulus in about 2¾ hours (5,000 ÷ 30 ÷ 60 = about 2.75 or, in SI terms, 1,500 ÷ by 9 ÷ 60 = about 2.75). The crew had better not let the gas rise this high with the well shut in, because serious trouble will occur.

Since the well is shut in, the gas cannot expand. Therefore, it retains the same pressure as it rises up the annulus. As the kick rises, the pressures at the top and bottom of the annulus increase. In figure 61 the casing pressure has increased to 3,100 psi (21,374.5 kPa) and the bottomhole pressure has increased to 8,500 psi (58,607.5 kPa).

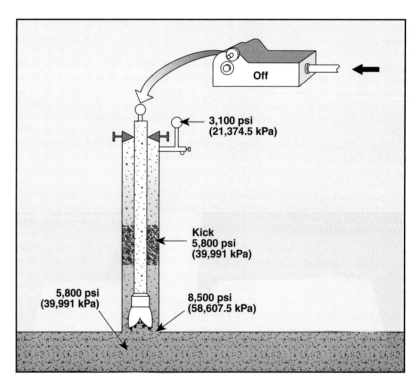

Figure 61.

The kick cannot expand. It still exerts 5,800 psi (39,991 kPa) of force. This force is applied in all directions. The kick pushes with 5,800 psi (39,991 kPa) of force both up and down. Pressure registering on the casing gauge results from the force of the gas minus the hydrostatic pressure of the mud between the gas bubble and the gauge. The bottomhole pressure is considerably higher, since it consists of the pressure of the kick plus the total hydrostatic pressure of the fluid below the kick. As the kick rises to the surface, the pressure at the casing gauge and throughout the well will continue to slowly increase.

One great danger throughout the whole process is the possibility of fracturing a formation, which can result in lost circulation and, possibly, an underground blowout. The blowout preventers could probably handle 5,800 psi (39,991 kPa) at the surface if the kick continued to rise, but the bottomhole pressure would rise to 11,200 psi (77,224 kPa or 77.2 MPa). A formation at some depth in the well would probably fracture long before the pressure actually got to such a high value.

Formation pressure remains at 5,800 psi (39,991 kPa). As the gas bubble rises, casing pressure becomes higher and higher. As stated earlier, the pressure exerted by the rising gas can become great enough to fracture a formation. Depending on the pressures involved, the formation may only fracture to the extent that kick fluids and drilling mud leak off into the formation relatively slowly. On the other hand, the formation could fracture so badly that all the fluids quickly leak into the formation. In this case, an underground blowout is underway.

The formation that fractures is usually just below the depth of the last casing string run into the well. The formation just below the casing is the weakest because it is usually the shallowest uncased formation. (The hydrostatic pressure of the fluids in shallow formations is less than in deeper ones.) To compound the problem, if the formation that fractures is just below the surface casing, the blowout can work its way around the outside of the casing and blow to the surface, creating a crater and a spectacular display of blowing fluids and fire.

So, we are dealing with a definite sequence of events. First, the kick takes place; then the well is shut in; the gas bubble starts to rise up the annulus causing an increase in pressure both above and below the bubble. This increase in pressure can fracture a formation and lead to partial or total lost circulation. Either can lead to a reduction in the hydrostatic pressure of the drilling mud. This in turn can lead to another kick. If the situation gets too far out of control, the well will have to be capped and abandoned; or worse, an underground blowout could occur, complicating things even further. So, the crew must begin to eliminate the kick in a relatively short period.

The key to safely handling a kick is to get the kick to the surface and out of the hole, while maintaining a constant pressure on the bottom of the hole that is equal to or slightly above formation pressure. The gas bubble must be allowed to expand and reduce in pressure but under controlled conditions. Therefore, mud must be vented from the well to allow room for the gas to expand.

The driller and rig supervisor (the personnel usually directly responsible for handling a kick) must ensure that the bottomhole pressure, which is hydrostatic plus remaining circulating pressure, remains equal to or slightly higher than the formation pressure. If bottomhole pressure is lower than formation pressure, further kicks occur. Taking more kicks makes it much harder to regain control of the well. Once the well is shut in, the situation stabilizes but only temporarily. A gas kick continues to rise. As it rises, it increases the pressure within the annulus. Too much pressure increase and lost circulation and fracturing could occur, leading to an underground blowout.

CIRCULATING CONSIDERATIONS

Drillers and rig supervisors have several ways to circulate the kick out of the well. This book goes through the general steps, and later examines the specific characteristics of two popular methods.

After the well is shut in and the pressure has temporarily stabilized, the kick must be circulated out of the well and the mud weight must be increased. The mud weight must be increased enough so that when it is circulated into the well it develops enough hydrostatic pressure to control the kicking formation. During these operations, the driller and supervisor must keep bottomhole pressure as constant as possible. If it drops too low, more kick fluids can enter the well. If it rises too high, a formation could fracture creating lost circulation.

Bottomhole pressure is held constant by (1) choosing a pumping rate (speed) and holding the pump at that speed while mud is circulated, and (2) by adjusting the choke opening (making it larger or smaller) as the mud and kick are circulated out of the well. Since the blowout preventers close in the top of the well, mud must be circulated out of the well through the choke. Opening the choke (making its opening larger) reduces the back-pressure held on the well. Closing the choke (making its opening smaller) increases the back-pressure. Figure 62 is a diagram of a well being circulated. The pump is on and is moving mud down the drill stem. Mud jets out of the bit and moves up the annulus. Note that the kick fluids also move up. The mud exits the well through the choke.

As the mud pump is started and the choke opened, mud and kick fluids move up the annulus. Mud is once again circulating through the well. When circulating, the small amount of circulating pressure needed to carry the mud to the top of the annulus increases the bottomhole pressure.

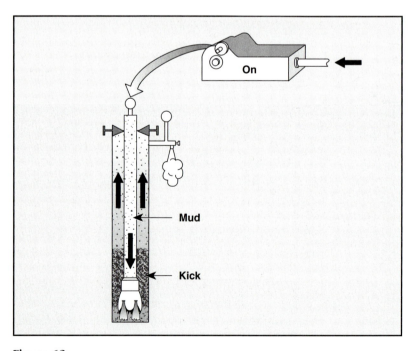

Figure 62.

The secret is to open the choke only enough to allow some of the mud to escape but not enough to reduce the bottomhole pressure and allow another kick. By adjusting the choke, the kick can be circulated up and out of the well while maintaining a constant bottomhole pressure.

Figure 63 shows a well shut in on a kick. The hydrostatic pressure of the mud in the drill stem just above the bit is 6,500 psi (44,817.5 kPa). Formation pressure is 7,000 psi (48,265 kPa). Formation pressure is therefore 500 psi (3,447.5 kPa) higher than the hydrostatic pressure. The well is successfully shut in and temporarily stabilized.

The next concern is maintaining a constant bottomhole pressure while circulating the kick out of the hole. So, mud starts to circulate at 2,000 psi (13,790 kPa) measured on the drill pipe gauge as the mud enters the drill stem. A pressure of 1,850 psi (12,756 kPa) is lost overcoming friction as the mud moves down the drill stem and out of the bit nozzles. The friction losses in the drill stem and nozzles leave 150 psi (1,034 kPa) circulating pressure underneath the bit to lift mud up the annulus. Without taking the back-pressure the choke holds on the well into account, the bottomhole pressure (hydrostatic plus circulating pressure) is 6,650 psi (45,851.5 kPa). This 6,650 psi (45,851.5 kPa) is not enough to keep out another kick, but by adjusting the choke, a high enough back-pressure can be maintained to prevent another kick. If the bottomhole pressure needs to be increased, the choke operator (usually the rig supervisor or toolpusher) closes in on the choke (reduces the size of the choke's opening). If the bottomhole pressure needs to be decreased, the choke operator opens the choke (increases the size of the choke's opening). Meanwhile, the driller keeps the pumping rate constant. Holding a constant pump rate while adjusting the choke keeps a steady amount of mud going into the well and the bottomhole pressure constant. The idea is to maintain just enough bottomhole pressure to prevent a kick without fracturing a formation.

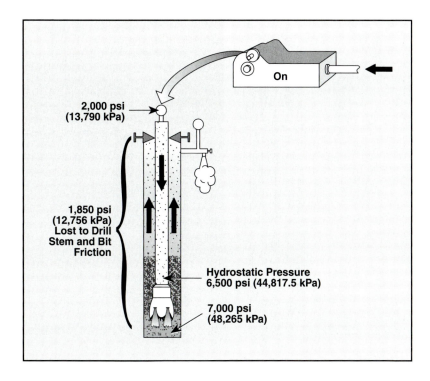

Figure 63.

If something needs to be checked or a calculation needs to be refigured, circulation can be stopped and the choke completely closed. Remember, however, that circulation should not be stopped for a lengthy period. The gas continues to rise up the well and increases the pressure on the casing shoe, which could lead to formation fracture below the shoe.

Figure 64 shows that the kick has been completely circulated out of the well. The BOPs are open and the well is full of mud that exerts 6,500 psi (44,817.5 kPa). However, formation pressure is still 7,000 psi (48,265 kPa). So, another kick is occurring. The BOPs can be left closed, the mud pump stopped, and the choke completely closed after the kick is circulated out of the well to prevent another kick. A kick can't occur, but neither can normal operations. The hydrostatic pressure must be increased to at least 7,000 psi (48,265 kPa) before normal operations can resume. Crew members can increase hydrostatic pressure by circulating heavier mud down the hole.

Some kick-killing methods circulate the heavier mud after eliminating the kick, and other methods increase the mud weight while venting the kick. The first method is simpler, but the second produces less pressure in the well and casing. The mud weight can be increased by mixing a weighting material such as barite in the mud and then circulating it down the hole.

Before examining how well-killing techniques work, two other points need to be examined—shut-in drill pipe pressure (SIDPP) and the initial circulating rate. These two items provide the information needed to find out the amount of pressure the kick is creating and, when circulating the kick from the well, what circulating pressure should be held on the drill pipe pressure gauge.

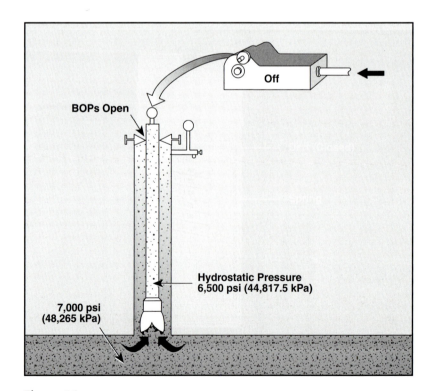

Figure 64.

INTRODUCTION TO WELL CONTROL

SHUT-IN DRILL PIPE PRESSURE (SIDPP)

When the bit is on bottom and drilling and a formation kicks, the kick usually enters the annulus and not the drill stem. The kick can only enter the drill stem through the small jet nozzles located in the bit. The kick follows the path of least resistance or lowest pressure. Since a considerable amount of circulating pressure is inside the bit (in fig. 65, 1,800 psi or 12,411 kPa), more pressure exists inside the bit than just below it in the annulus. So, when a kick occurs, the formation fluids flow up the annulus and not into the drill stem. After shutting in the well, the drill stem remains full of drilling mud. (Usually, if a kick occurs during a trip, the drill stem has kick fluids in it. The manual covers tripping later.)

The drill pipe pressure gauge normally registers the circulating pressure as mud enters the drill stem. In figure 66, the well is shut in and the mud pump is off; so the gauge should read 0 psi (0 kPa) circulating pressure. But the gauge in figure 66 reads 200 psi (1,379 kPa). This pressure must be coming from somewhere.

The 200-psi (1,379-kPa) reading represents the new formation pressure minus the hydrostatic pressure of the mud in the drill stem. The drill stem remains full of drilling fluid. This fluid does not compress very much; in fact, it is like hydraulic fluid. The pressure or force of the formation fluid pushes through the jet nozzles to the mud column in the drill stem. Because the mud column does not compress, the force transfers up the mud column and registers on the drill pipe gauge. This reading is called the shut-in drill pipe pressure (SIDPP).

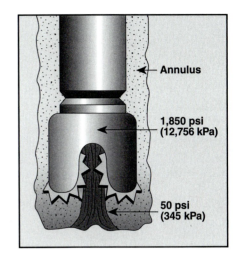

Figure 65.

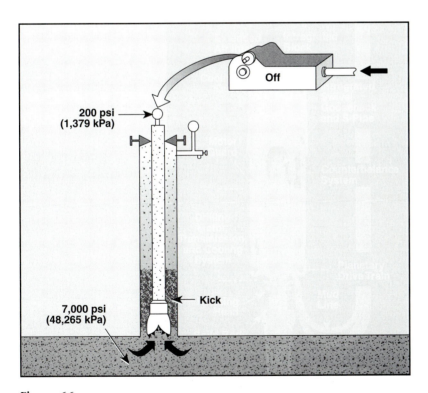

Figure 66.

Finding Kick Pressure

Shut-in drill pipe pressure provides valuable information for controlling the well. For instance, it indicates the difference between the hydrostatic pressure of the mud in the drill stem and the kicking formation pressure. Suppose, as in figure 67, the drill stem contains 12-ppg (1,438 kg/m³) mud and it is 10,000 feet (3,048 metres) deep. Mud that is 12 ppg (1,438 kg/m³) has a pressure gradient of 0.624 psi/ft (14.116 kPa/m). Therefore, the bottomhole hydrostatic pressure equals 6,240 psi or 43,026 kPa (pressure gradient times the depth). SIDPP is 250 psi (1,724 kPa). The shut-in drill pipe reading means that formation fluids are pushing upward with a force of 250 psi (1,724 kPa) greater than the hydrostatic pressure. The pressure of the kicking formation is determined by adding hydrostatic pressure and SIDPP. In this case, formation pressure is 6,490 psi (44,750 kPa).

Besides formation pressure, another important piece of information can be obtained from the SIDPP. Well killers need to know how much to increase the present mud weight to reach a new hydrostatic pressure high enough to kill the well. Formulas are available to determine the increase. In the English system, one formula is:

mud weight increase (ppg) = SIDPP (psi) ÷ TVD (ft) ÷ 0.052.

You may also see this formula expressed as:

mud weight increase (ppg) = SIDPP (psi) ÷ TVD (ft) × 19.23.

The second formula is like the first except that the result of the mud weight increase times SIDPP is multiplied by a constant rather than divided. The results are the same. In this manual, we'll divide by the constant 0.052.

In SI units, one formula is:

mud weight increase (kg/m³) = SIDPP (kPa) ÷ TVD (m) ÷ 0.0098.

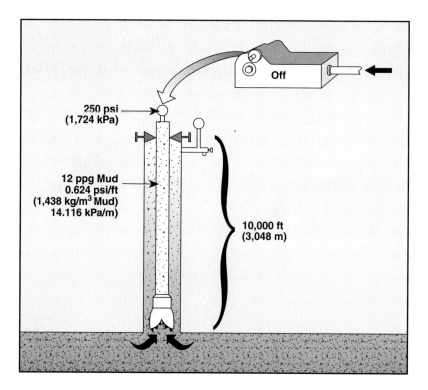

Figure 67.

You may also see this formula expressed as:

mud weight increase (kg/m³) = SIDPP (kPa) ÷ TVD (m) × 102.

The second formula is like the first except that the result of the mud weight increase times SIDPP is multiplied by a constant rather than divided. The results are the same. In this manual, we'll divide by the constant 0.0098.

As an example of determining mud weight increase in the English system, suppose SIDPP is 250 psi and the well's TVD is 5,000 feet. How much should the mud weight be increased to balance formation pressure? The answer is 250 ÷ 5,000 = 0.05 ÷ 0.052 = 0.96 = 1. The answer shows that the mud weight in use when the well kicked must be increased by 1.0 ppg to develop enough hydrostatic pressure to balance formation pressure. Thus, if 12-ppg mud was in use when the well kicked, it must be weighted up to 13 ppg to balance formation pressure.

As an example determining mud weight increase in the SI system, suppose SIDPP is 1,700 kPa and the well's TVD is 1,500 metres. How much should the mud weight be increased to balance formation pressure? The answer is 1,700 ÷ 1,500 = 1.13 ÷ 0.0098 = 115.3. The answer shows that the mud weight in use when the well kicked must be increased by 115.3 kg/m³ to develop enough hydrostatic pressure to balance formation pressure. Thus, if 1,400.0 kg/m³ mud was in use when the well kicked, it must be weighted up to 1,515.4 kg/m³ to balance formation pressure.

Figure 68 depicts another kicking well. It has a TVD of 10,000 feet (3,048 metres). SIDPP reads 750 psi (5,171 kPa). How much does the mud weight need to be increased in ppg to balance the kicking formation? The answer: 750 ÷ 10,000 = 0.075 ÷ 0.052 = 1.44 = 1.4. The mud weight must be increased 1.4 ppg to balance formation pressure. So, if a 9 ppg mud was in use, it must be weighted up to 10.4 ppg.

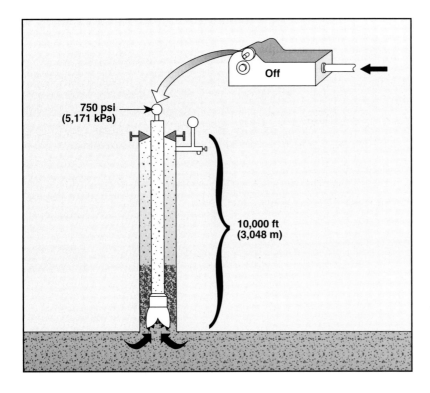

Figure 68.

How much does the mud weight need to be increased in kg/m³? The answer: 5,171 ÷ 3,048 = 1.70 ÷ 0.0098 = 173.5. The mud weight must be increased 173.5 kg/m³ to balance formation pressure. So, if a 1,078 kg/m³ was in use, it must be weighted up to 1,251.5 kg/m³.

Figure 69 shows one more kicking well. SIDPP is 450 psi (3,103 kPa). The well is 9,000 feet (2,743.2 metres) deep, and the old mud weight (the mud that is in the well when it kicked) is 9.0 ppg (1,078.4 kg/m³). What is the new mud weight (the weight of the mud required to kill the kick)? The answer is 450 ÷ 9,000 = 0.05 ÷ 0.052 = 0.96 = 1 ppg. The new mud weight is therefore 10.0 ppg. In SI units, the answer is 3,103 ÷ 2,743.2 = 1.13 ÷ 0.0098 = 115.3 kg/m³. The new mud weight is 1,193.7 kg/m³.

In summary, remember that SIDPP is important because the driller and supervisor use it to determine kick pressure. They can also use SIDPP to determine new mud weight—the mud weight needed to increase hydrostatic pressure enough to kill the well.

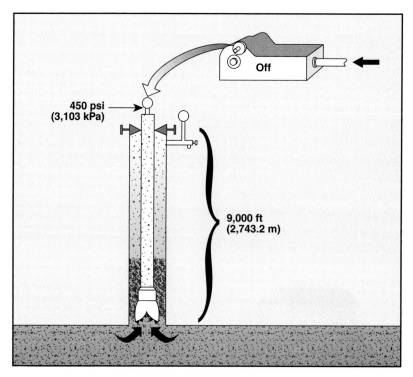

Figure 69.

Kill Rate

During most well-killing procedures, drilling mud should be circulated at a constant rate. In other words, the pump must be run at a constant speed. If the circulation rate changes, the downhole pressure also changes. With most well-control methods, downhole pressure is controlled by adjusting the choke and not the mud pump's speed. So, if a well-control operator sets a pump at 30 strokes per minute (spm), the pump circulates the same amount of mud each minute at the same pressure, as long as the pump's speed (spm) does not change.

TABLE 1

SPM	30	34	42	49	55	60
Pressure, psi (kPa)	800 (5,516)	1,000 (6,895)	1,500 (10,343)	2,000 (13,790)	2,500 (17,238)	3,000 (20,685)

Table 1 shows one particular pump's pressure at various strokes per minute (spm). Notice that as speed increases, so does pump pressure. The same thing happens to your water hose when you turn the faucet higher. If you keep the nozzle set at the same opening but increase the amount of water coming into the hose, the pressure of the water inside the hose increases.

In table 1, when this example pump runs at 30 spm, it puts out 800 psi (5,516 kPa). To increase the pressure to 3,000 psi (20,685 kPa), the pump's speed has to be increased to 60 spm. Rather small changes in the pump's speed can result in rather large changes in pressure. When circulating a kick, the well-control operator has to determine at what speed, and therefore at what pressure, to run the pump. Whatever speed is selected, this speed is called the kill rate.

Under most circumstances, when circulating the kick out or circulating heavier mud into the well, it is necessary to run the mud pump at a constant speed—the kill rate. With the pump running at a constant speed, the operator controls pressure in the well by adjusting the size of the choke opening. Normally, the kill rate is set at about one-quarter to one-half the pump's speed. Further, several kill rate speeds are usually chosen, in case one speed is unsuitable for well conditions. Kill rate speeds are lower than normal drilling speeds. By running the pump at a lower speed, crew members are given plenty of time to mix and add mud-weight material, usually barite. The lower speed also reduces the strain on the pumps and allows a safety factor when circulating the kick out. Kill rates are routinely selected and checked during normal operations before a kick may occur, thus eliminating one variable in the well-control procedure when a kick does occur. Usually, at least once a tour, the driller reduces the pump speed to the preselected kill rates and records the circulating pressure that registers on the drill pipe pressure gauge. This reading is called the kill-rate pressure.

Kill-Rate Pressure

The kill-rate pressure, sometimes abbreviated as KRP, is the circulating pressure indicated on the drill pipe pressure gauge with the mud pump speed set at a preselected kill rate. As an example, suppose that the pump speed, when drilling under normal conditions, is 95 spm. At 95 spm, the pump moves mud at a rate of 418 gallons per minute (gpm) or 1.6 cubic metres per minute (m³/min) at a pressure of 2,750 psi (18,961 kPa). This pressure is shown on the drill pipe pressure gauge.

At reduced kill-rates, the amount of fluid the pump moves and the pressure at which it moves it drops. For instance, at a kill-rate speed of 50 spm, a pump may move mud at a volume of 250 gpm (0.95 m³/min), at a kill-rate pressure of 900 psi (6,205.5 kPa). At 40 spm, the volume drops to 200 gpm (0.76 m³/min), and the kill-rate pressure is 750 psi (5,171 kPa). Finally, at 30 spm, the volume goes down to 150 gpm (0.57 m³/min), and the kill-rate pressure is 600 psi (4,137 kPa). It is not so much the volume that the pump moves as it is the reduced circulating pressure that concerns the well-control operator.

Remember that the pressure the drill pipe pressure gauge (fig. 70) registers depends on the situation. First, when drilling under normal conditions, the gauge registers normal circulating pressure. When the pump is shut down, and no kick has intruded, the gauge registers zero. Second, if the well has kicked, the gauge reflects the difference between hydrostatic pressure and the pressure of the kicking formation after the well is shut in and the mud pump is shut down. With the pumps off and the well completely closed on a kick, the pressure that shows up on the drill pipe pressure gauge is called shut-in drill pipe pressure, or SIDPP. And third, when the BOPs are closed, the choke is open, and the pump is operating at the kill rate, the gauge registers initial circulating pressure, which is sometimes abbreviated as ICP.

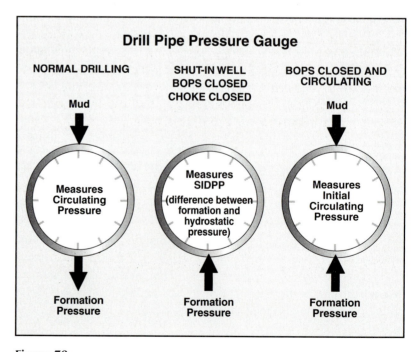

Figure 70.

Initial Circulating Pressure

Initial circulating pressure is the pressure the pump puts out at the reduced circulating rate (the kill rate), plus SIDPP. It is called initial circulating pressure because it changes later, when kill-weight mud is pumped down the drill stem to kill the well. (When pumping kill-weight mud, the well-control operator reduces SIDPP to final circulating pressure. More about final circulating pressure later.) By checking SIDPP, the operator knows how much higher the formation pressure is than the hydrostatic pressure. Because the kill rate was selected and recorded before the well kicked, the operator also knows how much pressure it produces.

SIDPP and kill-rate pressure enable a well-control operator to begin circulating the mud and kick out of the well after it is closed in. The operator simultaneously opens the choke and starts the pump. By opening the choke as the pump comes up to kill-rate speed, the operator reaches initial circulating pressure, which the drill pipe pressure gauge shows. If SIDPP goes higher or lower than the initial circulating pressure, then the operator adjusts the size of the choke's opening but keeps the pump speed constant at the preselected kill rate. By maintaining constant pump speed, and adjusting initial circulating pressure displayed on the drill pipe pressure gauge, the operator keeps bottomhole pressure constant, which is vital to most well-control procedures. All of this information can be converted into the following formula:

kill-rate pressure (KRP) + SIDPP = initial circulating pressure (ICP).

The kill-rate pressure is the amount of force necessary to move the mud through the well with the pump operating at the kill rate. SIDPP is the difference between the hydrostatic and the formation pressure. As an example, suppose that SIDPP is 250 psi (1,725 kPa) and the kill-rate pressure is 1,200 psi (8,275 kPa) at 35 spm. What is the initial circulating pressure? The answer is 250 (1,725) + 1,200 (8,275) = 1,450 psi (10,000 kPa). In this case, the well-control operator will begin circulating the kick out of the well using a pump speed of 35 spm while maintaining 1,450 psi (10,000 kPa) on the drill pipe pressure gauge. The job from then on consists of keeping the pump running at 35 strokes per minute and adjusting the choke to maintain the initial circulating pressure on the drill pipe gauge. As mentioned earlier, when heavier mud starts to circulate, the reading changes, but we will deal with that shortly. For now, let's take a closer look at a simple well-killing method.

THE DRILLER'S METHOD

The driller's method is a widely used well-killing procedure. It consists of two separate and complete circulations. The first circulation pumps the kick out of the well. While the well remains shut in, the weight of the mud in the tanks is increased to the weight required to control the formation pressure. The second circulation then pumps the heavier mud into the well to increase the hydrostatic pressure. The mud pump operates at a constant speed throughout both circulations, and the well-control operator controls bottomhole pressure by adjusting the choke. Once the second circulation is completed, pumping stops and a check of SIDPP and shut-in casing pressure (SICP) is made. If both gauges show zero, the BOP can be opened and normal drilling operations resumed. If both gauges do not register zero, then the new SIDPP and SICP are recorded and the process repeated. The driller's method does not require complex calculations or graphs and allows a well-control operator to use straightforward and uncomplicated techniques. For these reasons, many contractors and operators prefer the driller's method to others.

Let's follow a well-control operator as a kick is taken and eliminated with the driller's method. Figure 71 is a schematic of what is happening.

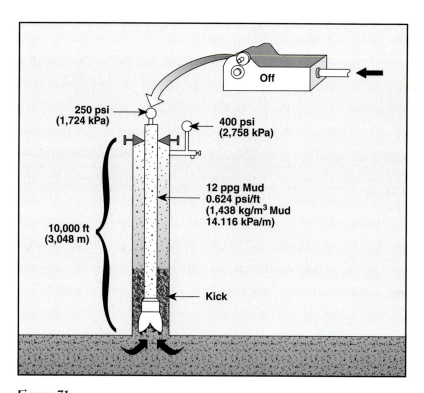

Figure 71.

The depth of the well is 10,000 feet (3,048 metres). The mud weight is 12 ppg (1,438 kg/m³). The well is shut in and the SIDPP is 250 psi (1,724 kPa). Casing pressure is 400 psi (2,758 kPa). Once the mud pump has reached the kill rate, it is not necessary to be too concerned with the casing pressure since most actions are based on the pressure registering on the drill pipe pressure gauge. The casing pressure gauge should, however, be checked periodically to be sure it does not rise above the pressure limits of the casing shoe.

As for pressure limits on the formation at the casing shoe, this limit should be determined and recorded before a kick occurs. Fracture pressure of the formation below the casing shoe can be determined by pumping mud into the well after the casing is run and cemented to the point where the formation begins to fracture. The pressure at which fracture just begins to occur is recorded and used for reference should the well kick.

When a kick is taken while the bit is on bottom and drilling, and the kick is gas or mostly gas, shut-in casing pressure (SICP) is higher than SIDPP. SICP is higher than SIDPP because the drill stem is full of drilling mud that is uncontaminated by the kick. The casing annulus, on the other hand, is contaminated by the kick. If the kick is gas, it expands when it enters the annulus and therefore exerts more pressure on the casing gauge than the clean mud in the drill stem exerts on the drill pipe gauge.

Referring to figure 71, note that the hydrostatic pressure is 6,240 psi (43,026 kPa) because the pressure gradient of 12-ppg (1,438-kg/m³) mud is 0.624 psi/ft (14.116 kPa/m) and the well is 10,000 feet (3,048 meters) deep. Therefore, $0.624 \times 10,000 = 6,240$ psi ($14.116 \times 3,048 = 43,026$ kPa). The mud weight needs to be increased to 12.5 ppg (1,496 kg/m³) before the second circulation because the mud weight increase equals SIDPP (psi) ÷ TVD (ft) ÷ 0.052 added to the old mud weight (ppg), which is 250 psi ÷ 10,000 feet = 0.025 ÷ 0.052 = 0.48 = 0.5 ppg; thus, 12 + 0.5 = 12.5 ppg. In SI units, the increase equals SIDPP (kPa) ÷ TVD (m) ÷ 0.0098 added to the old mud weight (kg/m³), which is 1,724 kPa ÷ 3,048 metres = 0.57 ÷ 0.0098 = 58.16 = 58 kg/m³; thus, 1,438 + 58 = 1,496 kg/m³. Finally, the well-control operator needs to determine the initial circulating pressure and the operator will be ready to circulate the kick out.

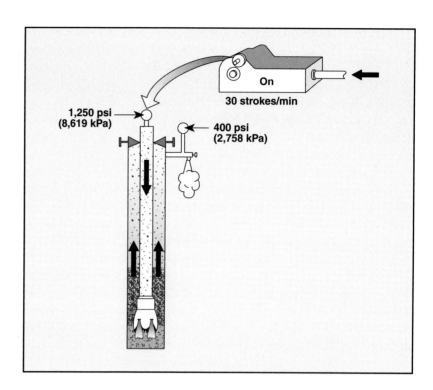

Figure 72.

Previously, the driller recorded the mud pump kill rate at 30 strokes per minute (fig. 72), which produced a kill-rate pressure of 1,000 psi (6,895 kPa) on the drill pipe pressure gauge. The 1,000 psi (6,895 kPa) was the amount of force used to circulate the mud through the mud system before the kick occurred. But the kick creates another 250 psi (1,724 kPa) of force that must be overcome. So the initial circulating pressure is the original kill-rate pressure of 1,000 psi (6,895 kPa) plus the SIDPP of 250 psi (1,724 kPa) for the kick, making a total of 1,250 psi (8,619 kPa).

Now that all the calculations are done, killing the kick can begin. The well-control operator starts the mud pump and at the same time opens the choke. To keep bottomhole pressure constant while opening the choke and starting the pump, the operator observes SICP and, in this case, keeps it at 400 psi (2,758 kPa) by manipulating the choke control as the pump is brought up to the kill rate. Maintaining 400 psi (2,758 kPa) casing pressure keeps bottomhole pressure constant to prevent more kick fluids from entering the well and to prevent a formation from fracturing from pressure too high.

After the mud pump reaches the kill rate, the operator switches attention to SIDPP and bases choke adjustments on the drill pipe pressure gauge readings. When the pump is operating at the kill rate, the drill pipe gauge must, in this example, register 1,250 psi (8,619 kPa) at all times while mud and the kick are being circulated out through the choke. If the pressure falls below 1,250 psi (8,619 kPa), the choke is closed to increase the pressure. If the pressure rises above 1,250 psi (8,619 kPa), the choke is opened to lower the pressure.

Figure 73 shows the well after some time has passed. The kick has moved up the annulus and has increased somewhat in volume. Also, SICP has increased to 700 psi (4,827 kPa). This increase is normal because, as the gas goes up the annulus, it exerts more pressure at the top of the

INTRODUCTION TO WELL CONTROL

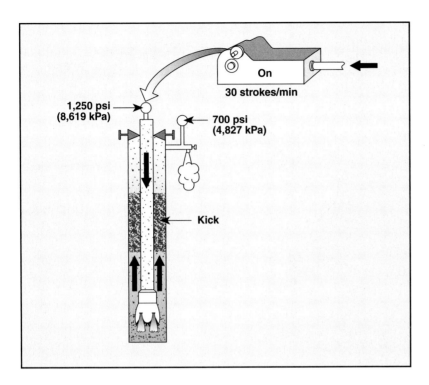

Figure 73.

well. Everything is okay at this point, because the drill pipe pressure is still 1,250 psi (8,619 kPa), and the mud pump is being maintained at a constant 30 spm. Also, while not shown in figure 73, the level (volume) of mud in the mud tanks rises and the gas rises and expands on its way up the annulus. This increase in tank volume is normal while a gas kick is being circulated up the annulus.

Figure 74 shows the well after more time has gone by. Note SIDPP. It has gone up to 1,400 psi (9,653 kPa). SIDPP is too high and should

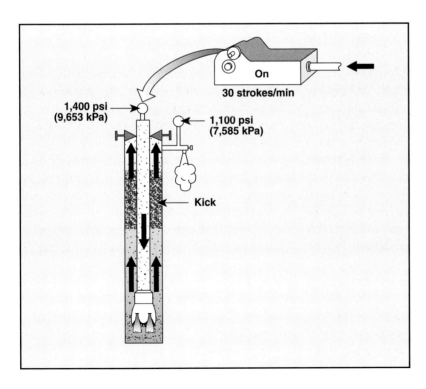

Figure 74.

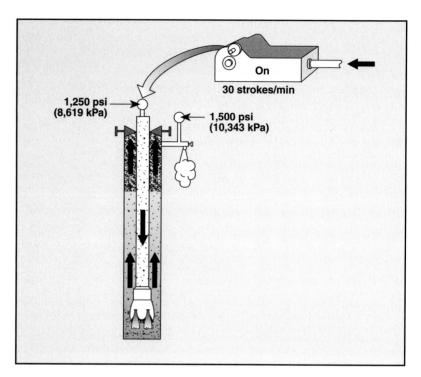

On

30 strokes/min

1,250 psi
(8,619 kPa)

1,500 psi
(10,343 kPa)

Figure 75.

be reduced to 1,250 psi (8,619 kPa). The high SIDPP indicates that bottomhole pressure has been allowed to get too high and it is possible to fracture a formation. Because the mud pump's speed is still 30 spm, to correct the situation, the well-control operator opens the choke a little until SIDPP gets back to 1,250 psi (8,619 kPa). Figure 75 shows the well in stable condition again. One thing to keep in mind: choke adjustments take about 1 second per linear foot (about 3 seconds per linear metre) down the drill stem and back up the annulus. Thus, for a 10,000-foot (3,048-metre) well, a 20-second delay occurs between a choke adjustment and the change on the drill pipe pressure gauge. To get around the delay, a well-control operator can use the casing pressure gauge to make choke adjustments. In this example, the operator needs to reduce SIDPP by 150 psi (1,034 kPa). So, the operator adjusts the choke to immediately reduce SICP by 150 psi (1,034 kPa). This change shows up on the drill pipe pressure gauge about 20 seconds later.

Casing pressure continues to rise until the kick is vented. As long as SICP does not rise above the amount of pressure that fractures the formation below the casing shoe, rising SICP is not a problem, because as the gas comes up, hydrostatic pressure on it is reduced and its pressure rises. The main concern is maintaining constant pressure on the drill pipe gauge. Once the kick is completely vented, SICP should drop to the pressure that was the original SIDPP, which is 250 psi (1,724 kPa), in this example. In other words, after the kick is completely circulated out of the well, SIDPP and SICP should read the same.

After the kick is completely vented and the casing pressure has fallen to the original SIDPP, the mud pump should be stopped and the choke completely closed. Crew members can now add a weighting material (usually barite) to the mud in the mud tanks to increase its weight to the required amount. In this case, the old mud weight of 12 ppg (1,438 kg/m3) is increased by 0.5 ppg (58 kg/m^3). The new mud weight of 12.5 ppg (1,496 kg/m^3) exerts enough hydrostatic pressure to hold back the higher formation pressure and prevents more kicks.

To begin pumping the new mud, the well-control operator opens the choke and slowly brings the pump up to kill-rate speed, while adjusting the choke to maintain SICP, which is now the same as SIDPP. When the pump reaches kill-rate speed, the operator adjusts the choke to continue to hold SICP constant as the new, heavy mud fills the drill stem. The operator uses SICP to maintain pressure because SIDPP falls as the new mud goes down the drill stem. SIDPP falls because the new mud creates more hydrostatic pressure than the old mud. This higher hydrostatic pressure offsets the pressure exerted by the formation. Once the heavier mud fills the drill stem, the operator switches his attention to SIDPP, which is now lower than it was before the heavy mud killed the pressure in the drill stem. In fact, if all the calculations are correct, SIDPP should be at the kill-rate pressure (1,000 psi or 6,895 kPa in this example) since the drill stem is full of new mud. With the drill stem full of new mud, the operator holds SIDPP constant with the choke until the new mud completely fills the annulus and goes out the return line to the tanks.

Once the heavier mud fills the drill stem and annulus, the operator stops the pumps, completely closes in the well, and checks to see if both SIDPP and SICP read zero. If they do, then the BOPs can be opened and normal operations continued. If not, then the well has kicked again and kill procedures must be repeated.

Most operators and contractors require that rig personnel use a written guide to steer them through a well-control procedure. Often called kill sheets, figure 76 is a sample of a simple kill sheet for the driller's method in English units of measure. Notice that it is divided into six parts, which help guide personnel through the procedure. Section one is for prerecorded information—items that need to be written down before a kick ever happens. This kill sheet has spaces for casing size and depth, its rated burst pressure, and the maximum allowable SICP. SICP above the maximum allowable fractures the formation below the casing shoe, which could lead to an underground blowout. (What to do if SICP goes too high is not discussed in this manual, but it involves bleeding the casing pressure through the choke as heavy mud is pumped into the well in stages. See the PETEX book, *Practical Well Control* for more information.) The kill sheet also has spaces for normal circulating pressure and pump rate as well as spaces for three kill-rate pressures and rates. Sections two through six have spaces for personnel to fill in when a kick occurs and provides simplified instructions for the driller's method.

WELL-CONTROL KILL SHEET
DRILLER'S METHOD (SIMPLIFIED)

1. **Prerecorded information**
   a. Casing size _____ in. Depth _____ ft
   b. Rated casing burst _____ psi
   c. Maximum allowable SICP _____ psi
   d. Normal circulating pressure _____ psi
      Normal circulating pump rate _____ spm
   e. Reduced circulating pressures (kill rates)
      (1) _____ psi   Rate _____ spm
      (2) _____ psi   Rate _____ spm
      (3) _____ psi   Rate _____ spm

2. **Stop pump and close well completely.**
   a. SIDPP _____ _____ psi
   b. SICP _____ _____ psi
   c. Mud weight _____ _____ ppg
   d. True vertical depth ____ _____ feet
   e. Pit gain _____ _____ bbl
   f. Circulating time, surface to bit _____ min

3. **Set circulating rate and pressures to remove kick.**
   a. Start pump and open choke. Choke pressure initially should be SICP. Maintain this pressure while the pump is brought up to kill-rate speed.
   b. Adjust choke to maintain SIDPP plus kill-rate speed.
   c. Reduced circulating SIDPP _____ psi
      Rate _____ spm
   d. Maintain pump rate constant at reduced speed and maintain SIDPP constant. If SIDPP increases, open choke. If SIDPP decreases, close choke. Use SICP to adjust choke to avoid time lag on SIDPP.
   e. When well is free of kick, stop pump and close in well. At this time, annulus and drill pipe pressure should be same as original SIDPP.
   f. Record new SICP _____ _____ psi

4. **Calculate mud density to kill well.**
   Calculate mud weight increase (MWI) from information recorded in step 2.

   $$MWI = SIDPP \div TVD \div 0.052$$

5. **Increase surface mud to required density.**
   If mud weighting can be done in separate tank, start it at step 3.

6. Set circulating rate and pressures to kill well.
   a. Start pump and open choke. Pressure initially held on well by choke should be SICP (3f); maintain this pressure while the pump speed comes up to kill-rate speed.
   b. Adjust choke to hold SICP until drill stem is full of new, heavier mud.
   c. After drill stem is full of new mud, record SIDPP and hold pump rate and SIDPP constant by varying choke opening until annulus is filled with new mud.
   d. When new mud reaches the surface, bleed off choke pressure (if any); stop circulating and check well for flow.

Figure 76.

The kill sheet on your rig may not look anything like the one in figure 76, but it gives you an idea of a simple one.

In review, the driller's method consists of two major steps. First, after shutting in the well, the kick is circulated out. During this process, the mud pump is run at a constant speed and the bottomhole pressure adjusted by opening or closing the choke. If the bottomhole pressure increases significantly, lost circulation may result. If the bottomhole pressure decreases significantly, another kick might occur.

The second major step in the driller's method consists of increasing the mud weight and, therefore, the hydrostatic pressure and pumping the new mud into the well. The new mud prevents further kicks from occurring in that formation. After the original kick has been vented and the choke completely closed, the weight of the mud in the tanks is increased, usually by adding barite. After circulating the heavier mud down the drill pipe and back up the annulus, the well-control operator stops the pumps, shuts in the well completely, and checks SIDPP and SICP. If pressure is zero on both gauges, then the well is dead and normal drilling procedures can resume.

The driller's method requires only a few calculations and is easy to use. But, it does have some drawbacks. For instance, the kick is vented before circulating heavier mud down the hole, which may subject the well to a higher pressure in the annulus. This higher pressure could result in formation fracture or equipment failure. Also, since the technique requires two complete circulations, the well and equipment are subjected to higher pressures for longer periods than with other methods. Obviously, the faster a kick can be killed, the less danger of something going wrong. The trade-off becomes simplicity of operation versus higher pressures and longer delays.

THE WAIT-AND-WEIGHT METHOD

Another frequently used method of well killing is the wait-and-weight method (sometimes called the engineer's method). It subjects the well to less pressure, and the well can be killed faster than with the driller's method. The main drawback is that it involves more calculations, and the procedures are more complex.

The biggest difference is that the wait-and-weight method involves only one circulation while the driller's method needs two to kill the well. In the wait-and-weight method, kill-weight mud is pumped down the drill stem at the same time the kick is circulated up the annulus and out the choke. It has the name wait-and-weight, because, after detecting the kick, the crew shuts in the well and waits until the mud weight can be increased in the tanks. Then the kick is vented and the heavier mud circulated at the same time. Of course, the crew cannot wait too long (remember—that gas kick is going up the well even if it is shut in), so the wait-and-weight method is best suited for big rigs that can mix a lot of barite (or other weighting material) quickly.

Although the wait-and-weight method involves additional calculations, they are not difficult once the steps involved are understood. First, we'll see how the increased mud weight affects the pressure readings. A little later, we'll look at how to vent the kick. For now, just keep in mind that both processes are occurring simultaneously.

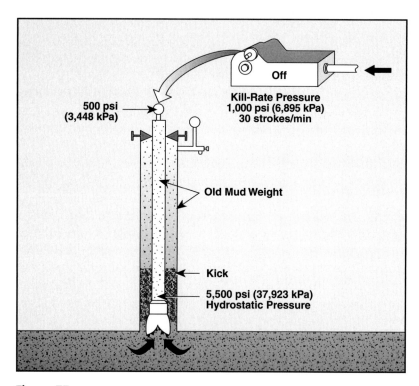

Figure 77.

In figure 77, the well is shut in and the mud pump is off. The predetermined kill-rate pressure is 1,000 psi (6,895 kPa) at 30 strokes per minute. SIDPP registering on the drill pipe pressure gauge is 500 psi (3,448 kPa). Hydrostatic pressure is 5,500 psi (37,923 kPa), so formation pressure is 6,000 psi (41,371 kPa). The drill stem is completely filled with mud at the old mud weight. The weight of the mud in the tanks has been increased to the required new weight.

In figure 78, the mud pump is started and the choke opened so that the heavier mud begins to flow down the drill stem. The drill pipe pressure gauge registered the initial circulating pressure of 1,500 psi or 10,343 kPa (kill-rate pressure + SIDPP), but it now reads 1,450 psi (9,998 kPa), a reduction of 50 psi (345 kPa). The mud column in the drill stem weighs more, so it exerts more hydrostatic pressure. As the difference between the new hydrostatic pressure and the formation pressure becomes less and less, SIDPP decreases. Remember that SIDPP is the difference between the hydrostatic and the formation pressures. Another kick has not occurred because bottomhole pressure is controlled with the choke.

In figure 79, the heavier mud is about halfway down the drill stem. The bottomhole hydrostatic pressure equals the pressure of the old mud plus the new, heavier mud. The addition of the heavier mud has increased the hydrostatic pressure at the well's bottom to 5,750 psi (39,646 kPa). But, what has happened to the drill pipe pressure? It has fallen to 1,250 psi (8,619 kPa). In the wait-and-weight method, this drop in SIDPP is to be expected because the heavy mud increases the hydrostatic pressure in the drill stem.

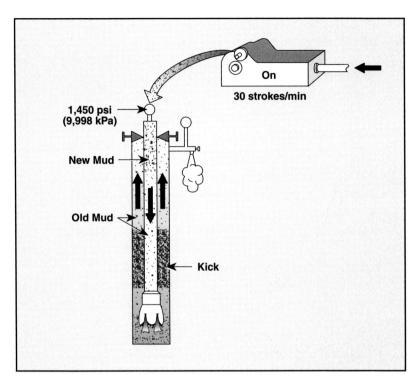

Figure 78.

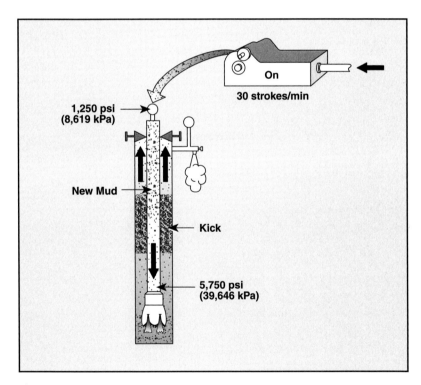

Figure 79.

The drill pipe pressure gauge is registering the kill-rate pressure and the difference between the hydrostatic and formation pressures. As heavy mud is pumped in, the difference between these two pressures becomes less. When the drill stem is full of heavier mud, hydrostatic pressure in the drill stem and formation pressure are equal. So the drill pipe gauge then only registers the kill-rate pressure of 1,000 psi (6895 kPa). If pumping is stopped and the choke is completely closed, SIDPP will register zero. (Remember that the drill stem is now completely full of heavier mud.)

In figure 80, the new, heavier mud has reached the bottom of the well and hydrostatic pressure equals formation pressure. But don't open the BOPs yet! The annulus still contains a mixture of the old, lighter mud and the kick. Therefore, the hydrostatic pressure in the annulus is considerably less than in the drill stem. If the BOPs were opened, another kick would flow up the annulus. The BOPs must be kept closed after venting the kick and the heavier mud circulated up and out of the annulus.

You may have recognized a problem with this whole procedure. The pressure registering on the drill pipe gauge decreases as new, heavier mud is pumped down the well. So, how are the choke adjustments determined as the kick is vented? With the driller's method, the initial circulating pressure was kept on the drill pipe gauge at all times while venting the kick. Simple, wasn't it? That won't work with the wait-and-weight method. What is needed is a plan or road map to indicate what the drill pipe gauge should register throughout the well-killing process. In short, a kill sheet is needed.

A kill sheet is a record of pertinent information and calculations. Let's plug some figures into the worksheet and see what happens. The purpose is to understand what is going on and not to actually teach all the steps involved in killing the well. Because this book is an introduction, we will use only the information necessary to fill in the sheet.

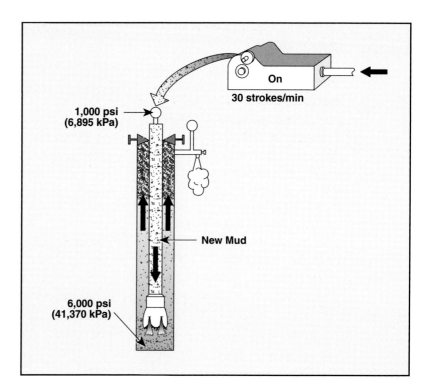

Figure 80.

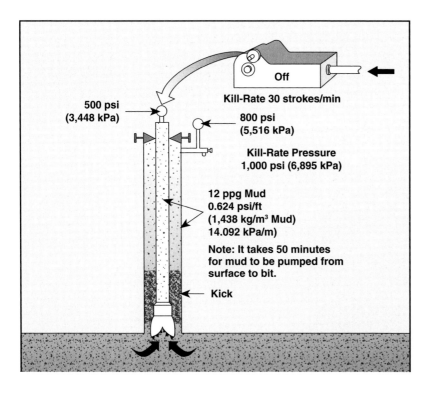

Figure 81.

Figure 81 is a schematic that shows a well kick. Figure 82 is a wait-and-weight method kill sheet. We'll fill in the information one step at a time. Step 1 is prerecorded information, the information the driller needs to get before the well kicks. In our simple example, the prerecorded information is the kill-rate pressure determined when the driller came on tour. So the blanks on the kill sheet are filled in as follows, using the information from figure 81.

1. *PRERECORDED INFORMATION*

    Kill-rate pressure at 30 strokes per minute is 1,000 psi (6,895 kPa).

    The information in step 2 is filled in immediately after shutting in the well.

2. *RECORDED AT TIME OF SHUT-IN*

    Circulating time, surface to bit: in this example well, it takes 50 minutes or 1,500 pump strokes. (If it takes 50 minutes for the mud to go from the surface to the bit, it also takes 1,500 strokes because 50 minutes × 30 strokes per minute = 1,500 strokes.) Surface-to-bit time and strokes are determined by knowing the length of the drill pipe and drill collars in feet or metres, the capacity of the drill pipe and collars in barrels per foot or cubic metres per metre, and how many barrels (cubic metres) of mud the rig pump puts out per stroke. Many tables and charts are available that show the capacity of drill pipe and drill collars and pump output per stroke.

    Shut-in drill pipe
    pressure (SIDPP)   =   500 psi (3,448 kPa)

    Shut-in casing
    pressure (SICP)   =   800 psi (5,516 kPa)

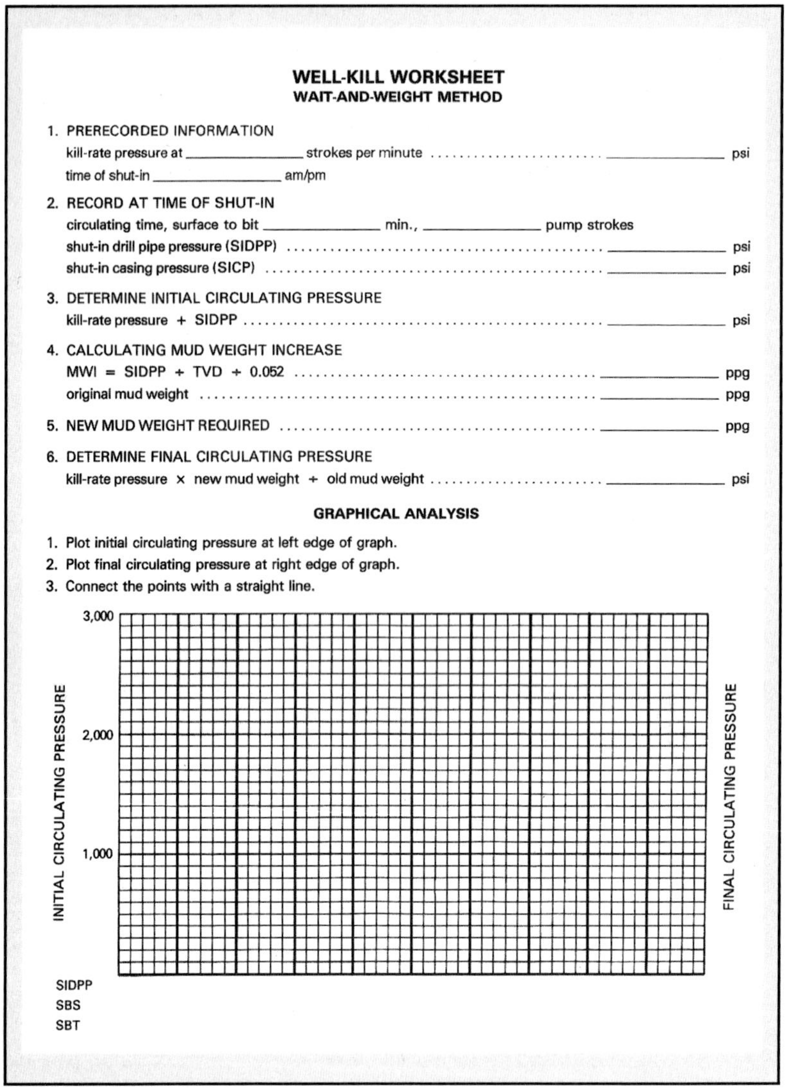

WELL-KILL WORKSHEET
WAIT-AND-WEIGHT METHOD

1. PRERECORDED INFORMATION
   kill-rate pressure at _____ strokes per minute .... _____ psi
   time of shut-in _____ am/pm

2. RECORD AT TIME OF SHUT-IN
   circulating time, surface to bit _____ min., _____ pump strokes
   shut-in drill pipe pressure (SIDPP) .... _____ psi
   shut-in casing pressure (SICP) .... _____ psi

3. DETERMINE INITIAL CIRCULATING PRESSURE
   kill-rate pressure + SIDPP .... _____ psi

4. CALCULATING MUD WEIGHT INCREASE
   MWI = SIDPP ÷ TVD ÷ 0.052 .... _____ ppg
   original mud weight .... _____ ppg

5. NEW MUD WEIGHT REQUIRED .... _____ ppg

6. DETERMINE FINAL CIRCULATING PRESSURE
   kill-rate pressure × new mud weight ÷ old mud weight .... _____ psi

GRAPHICAL ANALYSIS

1. Plot initial circulating pressure at left edge of graph.
2. Plot final circulating pressure at right edge of graph.
3. Connect the points with a straight line.

Figure 82.

Now figure initial circulating pressure (ICP). Initial circulating pressure is the amount of pressure that registers on the drill pipe gauge just before the heavier mud enters the top of the drill stem to be circulated down. Initial circulating pressure is equal to the kill-rate pressure plus SICP. At the same time the pump is started, the choke is opened and SICP is kept constant until the pump reaches kill-rate speed.

  3. *DETERMINING INITIAL CIRCULATING PRESSURE*
     Kill-rate pressure + SIDPP = 1,000 psi (6,895 kPa) + 500 psi (3,448 kPa) = 1,500 psi (10,343 kPa)

Before starting to circulate, the weight of the mud in the mud tanks must be increased. Steps 4 and 5 help to determine the new mud weight.

INTRODUCTION TO WELL CONTROL

4. *CALCULATING MUD WEIGHT INCREASE* (ppg, kg/m^3)

    SIDPP (psi) ÷ 0.052 ÷ TVD (feet)

    500 ÷ 0.052 = 9,615.385 ÷ 10,000 = 0.96 = 1 ppg

    SIDPP (kPa) ÷ 0.0098 ÷ TVD (metres)

    3,448 ÷ 0.0098 = 351,836.73 ÷ 3,048 = 115.43 = 115 kg/m^3

5. *NEW MUD WEIGHT REQUIRED* (ppg, kg/m^3)

    Old mud weight (ppg, kg/m^3) + weight increase (ppg, kg/m^3) = new mud weight (ppg, kg/m^3)

    12.0 + 1 = 13 ppg

    1,438 + 115 = 1,553 kg/m^3

Finally, final circulating pressure (FCP) needs to be calculated. Initial circulating pressure (ICP) registers on the drill pipe pressure gauge when the mud pump reaches kill-rate speed and just before the new mud starts down the drill stem. Final circulating pressure, which also registers on the drill pipe pressure gauge, occurs when the heavier mud reaches the bit (completely fills the drill stem). The two readings represent the highest and lowest pressure readings on the drill pipe gauge during circulation. Final circulating pressure is maintained while the new mud circulates up the annulus. Final circulating pressure can be determined with a simple formula.

6. DETERMINE FINAL CIRCULATING PRESSURE

    FCP = new mud weight ÷ old mud weight × kill-rate pressure

In our example well, the new mud weight is 13 ppg (1,553 kg/m^3) and the old mud weight is 12 ppg (1,438 kg/m^3). The kill-rate pressure is 1,000 psi (6,895 kPa). Thus, in English units, FCP = 13 ppg ÷ 12 ppg = 1.083 × 1,000 psi = 1,083 = 1,100 psi. (For practical purposes, we can round off.) In SI units, FCP = 1,553 kg/m^3 ÷ 1,438 kg/m^3 = 1.080 × 6,895 kPa = 7,446.6 = 7,447 kPa.

The last step is to put the initial and final circulating pressure on a graph. By drawing a line on the graph connecting the two pressures, it can be determined what the pressure should be at any time during the circulation.

With the driller's method, the initial circulating pressure is kept on the drill pipe pressure gauge while the kick is being vented, or circulated. Initial circulating pressure provided a guide for adjusting the choke. With the wait-and-weight method, initial circulating pressure provides only a starting point. Pressure on the drill pipe gauge decreases until the new mud completely fills the drill stem. With the drill stem full of kill-weight mud, the drill pipe pressure gauge reads final circulating pressure. Plotting initial and final circulating pressures on a graph provides the guide to correctly adjusting the choke.

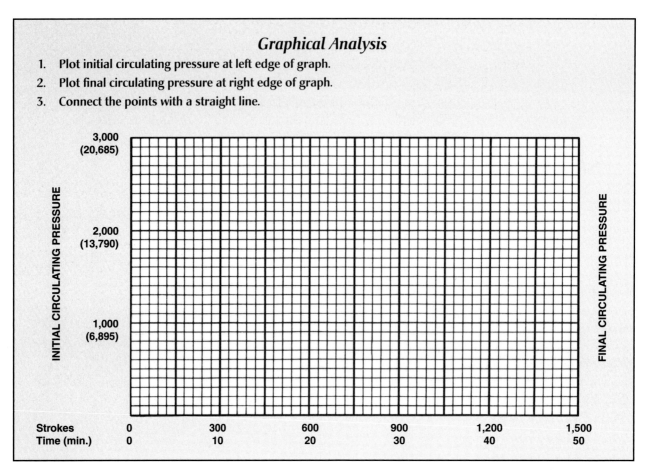

Graphical Analysis

1. Plot initial circulating pressure at left edge of graph.
2. Plot final circulating pressure at right edge of graph.
3. Connect the points with a straight line.

Figure 83.

Figure 83 is one type of graph used in the field. Such graphs are often found on the bottom of kill sheets, as in figure 82. The number of mud pump strokes and time in minutes it takes for the new mud to reach the bit is filled in along the bottom. This information is derived from step 2 on the worksheet.

The next step involves plotting the initial circulating pressure, which is 1,500 psi or 10,343 kPa (from step 3 on the worksheet). The left side of the graph shows different pressures on the horizontal lines. These lines of pressure range from 0 on the bottom of the graph to 3,000 psi (20,685 kPa) on the top of the graph. Going from 0 to 3,000 psi (20,685 kPa), are thirty horizontal lines, so each line going up the graph represents an increase of 100 psi (689.5 kPa).

Figure 84 is the graph with a line plotted from left to right. To plot the line, the initial circulating pressure of 1,500 psi (10,343 kPa) was found on the left side of the graph and a dot placed there. Then, the final circulating pressure of 1,100 psi (7,585 kPa) was found on the right side of the graph and a dot placed there. Finally, a straight edge was laid between the two dots and a line drawn to connect them. This line represents the pressure that must be maintained on the drill pipe pressure gauge during the circulation.

INTRODUCTION TO WELL CONTROL

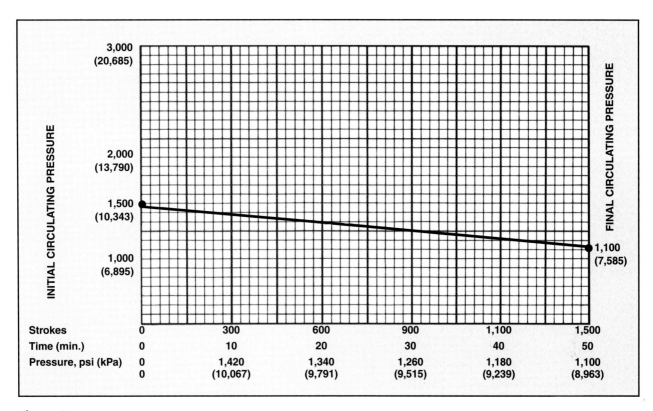

Figure 84.

By looking at the pump strokes or time listed on the bottom of the graph and then looking up at the line drawn on the graph, the correct pressure can be determined for any time during the circulation. For instance, after circulating for 10 minutes or 300 pump strokes, the pressure should have dropped to 1,420 psi (10,067 kPa) on the drill pipe gauge. If the gauge registers more or less than this, adjust the choke. At 20 minutes or 600 strokes, the gauge should register 1,340 psi (9,791 kPa). At 30 minutes the pressure should be 1,260 psi (9,515 kPa). At 40 minutes the pressure should be 1,180 psi (9,239 kPa). Finally, at 50 minutes and 1,500 strokes, the final circulating pressure of 1,100 psi (7,585 kPa) should be reached. Remember: if the gauge shows a higher or lower pressure, the choke must be adjusted.

Once the gauge registers the final circulating pressure of 1,100 psi, hold that pressure on the gauge until the heavier mud starts to flow out the choke. Once the new mud reaches the surface, the chances are good that the kick has been successfully killed and the BOPs can be opened. It is, however, a good idea to conduct a final flow test before opening the BOPs. Better safe than sorry.

Because exact pressures on a graph can be hard to determine, some operators and contractors do away with the graph and simply calculate the pressures in a table, as in table 2. In this example, the table is divided into ten steps after initial circulation. Some tables may use more or fewer steps. In table 2, the initial circulating pressure is 1,500 psi (10,343 kPa) and final circulating pressure is 1,200 psi (8,274 kPa).

The surface-to-bit time is 50 minutes and the surface-to-bit strokes is 800. (In other words, it takes 50 minutes and 800 strokes for the new mud to completely fill the drill stem.)

Also notice in table 2 that the pressure drop per division can be determined by subtracting final circulating pressure (FCP) from initial circulating pressure (ICP) and dividing the results by the number of divisions after ICP, ten in this case. So, in English units, $1{,}500 - 1{,}200 = 300 \div 10 = 30$ psi per division; or in SI units, $10{,}343 - 8{,}274 = 2069 \div 10 = 207$ kPa per division).

TABLE 2

Pressure = (ICP – FCP) ÷ 10 = _____ psi (kPa)/division

Time	0	5	10	15	20	25	30	35	40	45	50	Time
Pressure	ICP 1,500 (10,343)	1,470 (10,136)	1,440 (9,929)	1,410 (9,722)	1,380 (9,515)	1,350 (9,308)	1,320 (9,101)	1,290 (8,894)	1,260 (8,687)	1,230 (8,480)	FCP 1,200 (8,273)	Pressure
Strokes	0	80	160	240	320	400	480	560	640	720	800	Strokes

THE CONCURRENT METHOD

So far, the two most used methods of killing a kick have been covered: the driller's method and the wait-and-weight method. Another technique is the concurrent method (also called the circulate-and-weight method). It is similar to the wait-and-weight method, except the mud weight is not increased to its final weight and circulated all at once. In the wait-and-weight method, the well is shut in and crew members then increase the mud weight in the tanks the required amount. If a rig does not have the tank capacity to mix up the new mud weight all at once, and it is not desired to use the driller's method, then the concurrent method may be used.

In the concurrent method, the well is shut in, circulation begins immediately, and the weight of the mud is increased in increments, or steps, usually in tenths of a ppg, like 0.1 or 0.2 ppg, (10 or 20 kg/m³), as it circulates through the well. For example, if the mud weight needs to be increased by 1 ppg (120 kg/m³), and its original weight is 12 ppg (1,438 kg/m³), during the first circulation, crew members may raise the weight to 12.2 ppg (1,462 kg/m³); during the second circulation, they raise it to 12.4 ppg (1,486 kg/m³), and so on until 13 ppg (1,558 kg/m³) is reached. The concurrent method, like the wait-and-weight method, subjects the well to lower downhole pressure than the driller's method, thus reducing the risk of formation breakdown. But, it takes more calculations. For this reason, the concurrent method is not too widely used.

This section examines some typical well-control equipment designed to detect, handle, and eliminate kicks before they develop into blowouts. The intent is to familiarize you with the approximate locations and general functions of this equipment. You will receive instructions on the actual installation, operation, and maintenance of BOP equipment as part of your on-the-job training. The equipment is divided into the categories of blowout preventers, accumulators, equipment like control panels and drill stem valves, choke manifolds, mud-gas separators, and mud system equipment.

BLOWOUT PREVENTER STACKS

Most rigs have several blowout preventers stacked on top of each other. On land rigs and on jackup and platform rigs offshore, the stack is usually located directly under the rig floor (fig. 85). On offshore floating rigs, the stack is placed directly above the wellhead on the seafloor. The stack consists of several large valves capable of withstanding high pressure. Designed to shut in the well, the BOPs prevent a surface blowout from occurring.

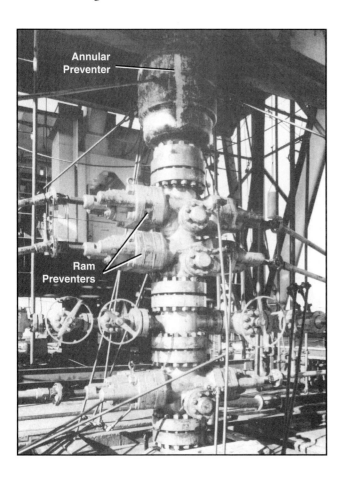

Annular Preventer

Ram Preventers

Figure 85.

PART IV
Well–Control
Equipment

Two general types of blowout preventers are available: annular and ram preventers. Moreover, several types of ram preventers are available, each designed to do a specific job. A common configuration for surface stacks is to place one annular preventer on top of the stack and several ram preventers below it. Some deepwater subsea stacks, on the other hand, may have two annular preventers mounted above the rams. Regardless of the stack's configuration, it is important for crew members to install the BOPs correctly. Stories abound about crews mounting one of the ram preventers upside down, for instance, and the rig's being lost when the BOP failed to work properly. If the preventers are not installed correctly, and if their parts are not installed correctly, the preventer could fail. What is more, the stack must be tested periodically and regularly to ensure that it will shut in the well efficiently and quickly.

Annular Preventers

First, let's look at an annular preventer (fig. 86). It gets its name because it is designed to close around the drill pipe, sealing off the annulus. An annular preventer has a large sealing element made of heavy-duty synthetic rubber (fig. 87). It resembles a doughnut. The drill pipe fits through the middle of the sealing element or doughnut hole. As the annular preventer closes, the sealing element seals tightly around the kelly, drill pipe, drill collars, tool joints, wireline, or anything else that might be in the hole (fig. 88). It can even seal an open hole (hole that has no pipe in it).

Once the preventer closes around the drill pipe or whatever is in the hole, the pipe can still be moved up or down through the preventer without the element's losing its pressure-tight seal. This action of moving pipe through a closed annular preventer is called stripping pipe, and is especially important if the kick takes place during a trip. In this case, the preventer shuts in the well and then allows the well-control operator to strip the pipe back to the bottom before circulation begins.

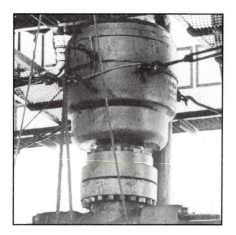

Figure 86.

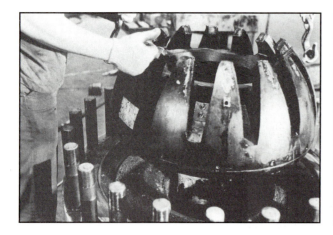

Figure 87.

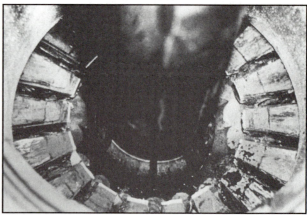

Figure 88.

You may have wondered how the BOP stack can hold back the tremendous pressure of a kick. Well, the stack is attached to the casing, which is cemented into the well. The casing acts like a huge anchor holding the blowout preventers in place. But what happens if a kick occurs before the surface casing is cemented into place? Even if the BOPs contain the kick, the pressure might be sufficient to fracture the surface formation and a blowout could occur underneath the rig floor. Using a special type of annular preventer called a diverter (fig. 89) can sometimes prevent a subsurface blowout. A diverter is a special type of annular preventer that, when closed around the drill pipe, has built-in valves that open. When the valves open, well flow is diverted inside large pipes away from the rig floor. If a shallow kick occurs, the driller closes the diverter and the kick is immediately vented, or diverted, away from the rig floor. Because the pressure cannot be contained, the gas is flared away from the rig. The diverter also must be tested on a regular schedule.

Ram Preventers

The second type of blowout preventer is called a ram preventer (fig. 90). A typical BOP stack includes different types of ram preventers, each designed to do a different job. It gets its name because it has two hydraulically operated sealing elements, or rams, installed inside a strong steel body. The rams are positioned in the BOP body so that one is on each side of the hole. As the preventer closes, the elements are forced, or rammed, together, sealing the hole. A regular pipe ram has half circles in the elements that fit exactly around a specific size pipe. In other words, if 5-inch (127.5-millimetre) drill pipe is in use, the rams must be sized to seal around 5-inch (127.5-millimetre) pipe.

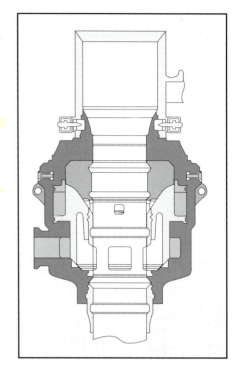

Figure 89.

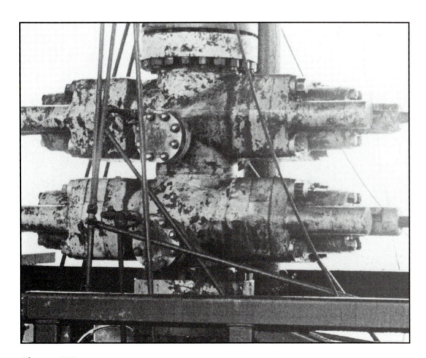

Figure 90.

A variable bore ram has special rams that can seal around a range of drill pipe sizes. For example, one type can seal around 3½-inch, 4-inch, and 4½-inch (88.9-millimetre, 101.6-millimetre, and 114.3-millimetre) pipe. If a kick occurs during a trip, the drill pipe can be stripped through the ram preventers, but it is easier to use the annular preventer.

The sealing elements on blind rams do not have the half circles. The two ram faces have elements that, when closed, seal off open hole. If someone accidentally closed the blind rams on drill pipe, the blind rams would crush the pipe and the hole would probably not be sealed effectively.

Shear rams (fig. 91), used mostly in subsea stacks, are similar to blind rams, but the elements are designed to cut, or shear, drill pipe and to seal the hole in an emergency. Offshore floating rigs often drill in areas where storms and hurricanes occur, so it is sometimes necessary for the rig to "shear and run." If necessary, the rig can suspend the drill stem in the hole by hanging it off on the pipe rams, then shear (cut) the pipe and move to a safe location. Later, the rig can come back and re-enter the hole by milling (grinding) out the closed shear rams and retrieving the drill stem.

In summary, blowout preventers are designed to shut in, or close off, the top of the well. There are two basic types of BOPs: annular and ram. Annular BOPs have a doughnut-shaped sealing element that closes around any size drill pipe, collar, or even an open hole. Regular pipe ram preventers need a different and specific size ram for each size drill pipe used. Variable bore pipe rams can seal around a range of drill pipe sizes. Blind rams are specifically designed to seal an open hole. Shear rams cut, or shear, any drill pipe as it seals the hole. A typical BOP stack will include one annular preventer and several ram preventers.

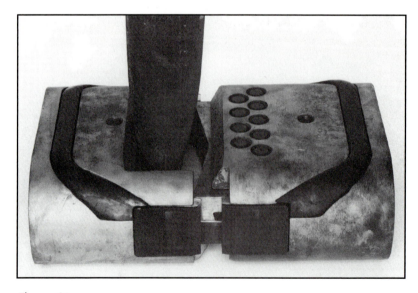

Figure 91.

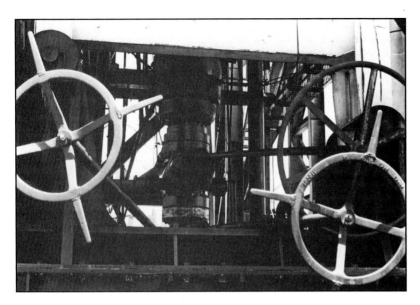

Figure 92.

Some ram blowout preventers can be operated either automatically or by hand. For example, the hand-wheels shown in figure 92 can be turned to close the ram preventers on a land rig. However, closing them by hand is slow, hard, and for emergencies only. The wheels can also be used to lock the preventers closed. Annular preventers and subsea preventers must be closed automatically. Subsea ram preventers and modern surface ram preventers are also automatically locked closed. Locking the preventers ensures that operating a special control valve can only open them. The automatic controls should be tested on a regular schedule to ensure that they are operating properly. In addition, periodic blowout drills should be conducted to teach the crew the proper procedures and each person's specific duties in case of a kick.

Accumulators

An important piece of equipment connected with the blowout preventer stack is the accumulator, or BOP operating unit (fig. 93). Although not a part of the stack itself, the accumulator supplies hydraulic pressure to close and open the blowout preventers. The system consists of several bottles (or cylinders) that contain hydraulic fluid at a pressure of up to 3,000 psi (20,685 kPa). By manipulating control valves on the accumulator, either directly or remotely from the rig floor, this pressurized fluid provides the force to operate both the annular and the ram preventers. When the accumulator valves are actuated to close or open the preventers, the stored pressure drops. As the bottles are depressurized, a small air pump automatically starts to repressurize them. Also, if the air system fails, most accumulators have an electric backup pump. The entire system should be checked daily for hydraulic leaks and fluid levels to insure it is operating correctly. Usually, none of the equipment is used very often, but it must be continually maintained and tested. Although it may be tempting to let equipment go unchecked, a lot is riding on its operating properly when a kick occurs.

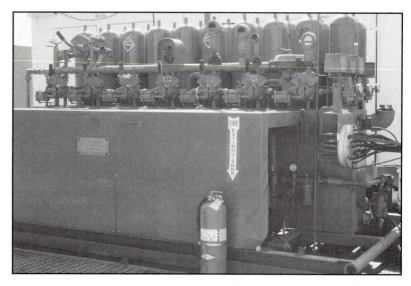

Figure 93.

ADDITIONAL BOP EQUIPMENT

Driller's Control Panel

Usually located on the rig floor near the driller's position, the driller's control panel provides remote-controlled operation of the BOPs (fig. 94). As mentioned earlier, the primary BOP controls are located on the accumulator, but the driller's control panel allows them to be operated from the rig floor. Sometimes, a second or third remote unit may be provided in places away from the rig floor and the accumulator. These additional remote panels may be needed if neither the rig floor nor the accumulator are accessible.

Kelly Cocks

The upper and lower kelly cocks are two valves installed above and below the kelly. The lower kelly cock is sometimes called a drill stem safety valve. The upper and lower kelly cocks provide a way of sealing the inside of the drill string. Sometimes a kick occurs during a trip when the drill string is off bottom. If the kelly can be stabbed, the lower kelly cock can be closed with a special wrench (fig. 95) to keep the kick from blowing out through the drill stem as well as to protect the rotary hose and swivel.

Drill Stem Safety and Gray Valves

If fluids are flowing out of the drill stem with such force that the kelly or top drive cannot be stabbed, a full-opening safety valve may be needed. With the valve inside the safety valve fully open, it can be placed into the flowing stream and over the drill stem opening. With the valve fully open, the pressure of the flowing fluids passes through the valve, which allows crew members to stab the device into the drill stem. With the safety valve stabbed and made up tightly, a special operating wrench is used to fully close the valve and stop flow. The kelly or top drive can then be stabbed into the drill stem.

Another type of valve that can be stabbed into the drill stem is a Gray valve (fig. 96). Named after one manufacturer of such valves, a Gray valve is used only when stripping pipe into the well. It is made up on top of a closed full-opening safety valve already made up in the drill stem. After the Gray valve's top assembly and actuating rod are removed, the check valve closes to keep intruded fluids in the drill stem from acting against the kelly or top drive, which is made up on top of the Gray valve.

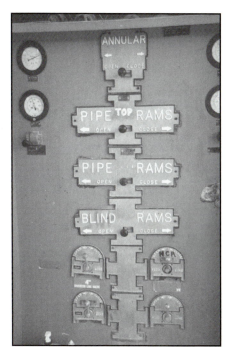

Figure 94.

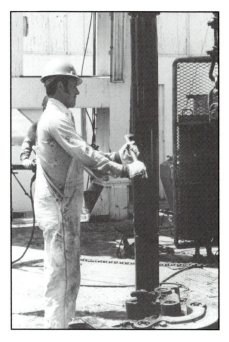

Figure 95.

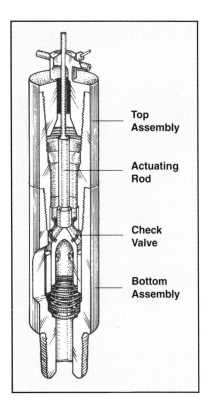

Figure 96.

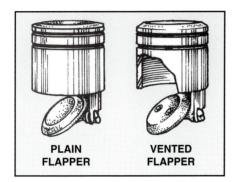

PLAIN FLAPPER **VENTED FLAPPER**

Figure 97.

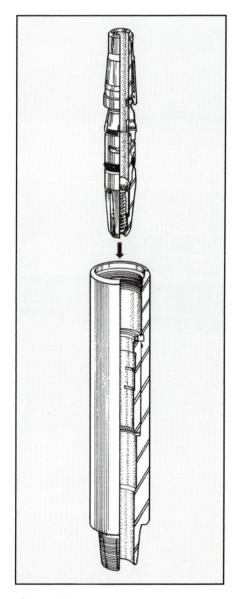

Figure 98.

Inside BOPs

The float valve (fig. 97) and drop-in valve, which is also called a pump-down valve (fig. 98), are inside blowout preventers (IBOPs). They seal the inside of the drill stem to prevent kick fluids from entering it. Float valves are installed in special drill stem substitutes (usually called subs, which are short sections of pipe that crew members install in the drill stem to perform a special function.) The sub that contains the float valve is usually installed above the bit or the drill collars. Float valves have a check valve, often in the form of a flapper, which opens when pressure is applied from above but closes against pressure from below. A vented flapper is available, which helps in obtaining SIDPP. Another type contains a dart valve (fig. 99), which a strong spring holds closed. Pump pressure from above overcomes spring pressure to open the valve during normal circulation.

Obtaining SIDPP when a float valve is installed calls for a special procedure, because the float valve closes off the inside of the drill stem and drill pipe pressure can therefore not be transmitted to the surface. Probably the best way to obtain SIDPP with a float valve is rig up a cement pump (a high-pressure, multicylinder pump that is used to pump cement into the well when running and cementing casing) to pump mud into the drill stem. The well-control operator then holds SICP constant with the choke while slowly pumping mud down the drill stem and keeping a close watch on SIDPP. When pressure builds enough to open the float valve, SIDPP will rise to a certain value and then stop rising. When SIDPP stops rising, the operator stops the pump and records SIDPP at the point where pressure stopped going up. This pressure should be SIDPP.

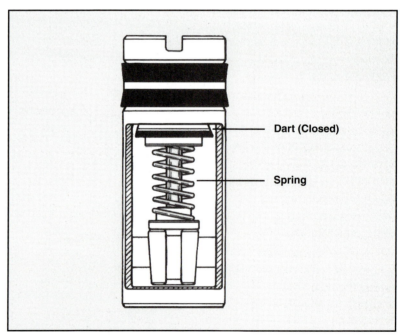

Dart (Closed)

Spring

Figure 99.

The mud pump can also be used to obtain SIDPP with a float valve installed in the drill stem. In this case, the operator keeps watch on SICP while pumping as slowly as possible. Pumping continues until the operator notes a rise in SICP. The pump is stopped and attention switched to the drill pipe pressure gauge. The pressure indicated on the gauge at this point should be SIDPP.

To use a pump-down check valve, crew members install a special landing sub in the drill stem, usually just above the drill collars, as they run the stem into the hole. Once the landing sub is made up, the check valve can be installed in one of three ways. If no fluids are flowing up the drill stem, a crew member simply drops the check valve into the stem when the kelly or top drive is disconnected from the stem. The kelly or top drive is then connected and the check valve is pumped down the stem to the landing sub.

If flow is occurring or is likely to occur, crew members can install the check valve through the lower kelly valve, or cock (also called a drill stem safety valve). With the lower kelly cock closed, crew members remove the kelly and place the check valve in the box of the kelly valve. Then they stab the kelly into the lower kelly valve and over the check valve. After crew members make up the kelly, they open the lower kelly valve and the driller pumps the check valve down the drill stem to the landing sub.

Finally, if a kick occurs during a trip and fluid is flowing from the drill stem, crew members can stab and make up a full-opening safety valve into the drill string. They then close the valve to stop flow. Next, they place the check valve into the box of the safety valve and make up the kelly over the safety valve. Pumping is started and the safety valve is opened to send the check valve down to the landing sub.

Top drives usually have two built-in IBOPs, which are similar to the upper and lower kelly cocks in a conventional kelly-drive system (fig. 100). The driller can open and close one of the IBOPs from a control panel on the operating console. Crew members operate the other IBOP manually. When closed, the IBOPs keep pressure inside the drill stem from acting on the top drive, rotary hose, standpipe, and mud pump.

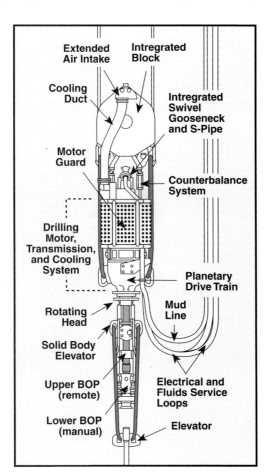

Extended Air Intake
Intregrated Block
Cooling Duct
Intregrated Swivel Gooseneck and S-Pipe
Motor Guard
Counterbalance System
Drilling Motor, Transmission, and Cooling System
Planetary Drive Train
Rotating Head
Mud Line
Solid Body Elevator
Upper BOP (remote)
Electrical and Fluids Service Loops
Lower BOP (manual)
Elevator

Figure 100.

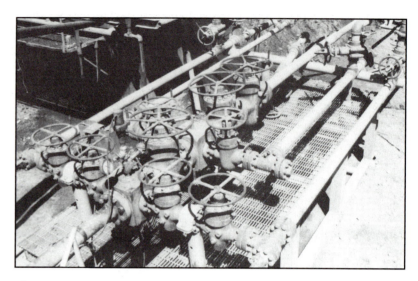

Figure 101.

CHOKE MANIFOLDS AND CHOKES

Closing the BOPs effectively shut in the top of the well. But once shut in, the kick must be circulated out of the well. Usually, the kick is vented out through the choke manifold (fig. 101). It consists of several pipes and valves. When a BOP on the wellhead is closed, the well-control operator directs the kick and mud in the annulus through a choke line installed below the BOP. A valve (often called an HCR valve) on the choke line is opened and circulation goes into the choke manifold. The choke manifold usually has several chokes. Often at least two of the chokes are adjustable and remote controlled (fig. 102). Others are manually adjusted, which means that a crew member has to be at the choke to adjust it. Manual chokes are mainly emergency backups. Adjustable chokes control the volume of fluid leaving the annulus and, therefore, the amount of pressure maintained at the bottom of the well.

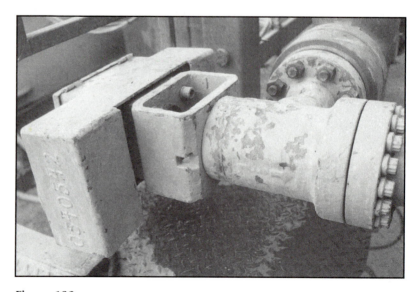

Figure 102.

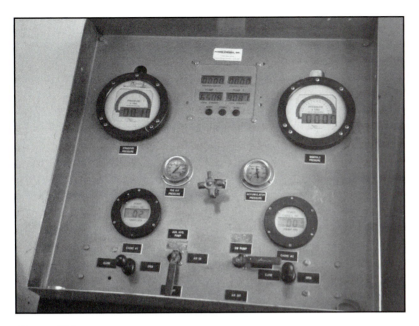

Figure 103.

Adjustable remote-controlled chokes have an opening that can be fully closed, fully open, or adjusted to any size from a position some distance from the choke, usually from a choke control panel on the rig floor (fig. 103). Besides a choke operating lever, many choke control panels also have drill pipe and casing pressure gauges, pump stroke counters, and other gauges and meters helpful in controlling and killing the kick. All the controls and valves should be tested or checked and lubricated periodically to ensure proper operation.

MUD-GAS SEPARATORS

After the mud and kick passes through the adjustable choke and choke manifold, the fluid is usually piped to a mud-gas separator (fig. 104). The separator, as its name implies, separates gas from drilling mud. After separation, the gas is vented and the mud goes back into the mud tanks to be recirculated. A special flare line carries the gas a safe distance away from the rig, where the gas is usually flared, or burned. Also, most contractors or operators install a bypass valve in the line carrying the gas and mud to the separator so that, if necessary, gas can be sent directly to the flare line without going through the separator. It may be necessary to bypass the separator when large volumes of gas are present. If the separator is not sized to handle the volume, then sending gas into it could damage or destroy the separator. The mud-gas separator consists of a series of baffle plates and requires little maintenance except periodic checking for leaks.

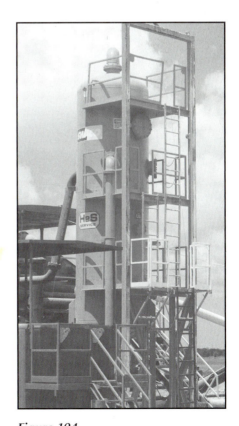

Figure 104.

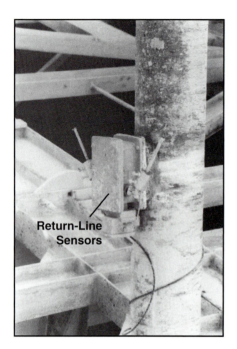

Figure 105.

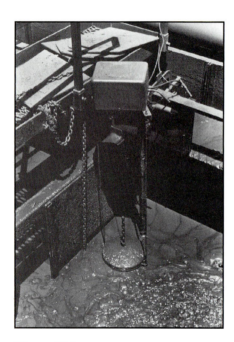

Figure 106.

MUD SYSTEM EQUIPMENT

As mentioned earlier, the mud returning up the annulus provides one of the best indications of an impending kick. A number of specialized pieces of equipment are used to detect any changes in the mud flow rate, volume, or physical composition.

Flow Indicators

The flow indicator senses and measures the rate of flow of the mud returning from the annulus (fig. 105). One type consists of a paddle located in the flow line, a device that senses the paddle's movement as the mud flows past it, a gauge or computer readout on the driller's console, and an audible and visual alarm. To use the system the driller sets the sensor to recognize a normal rate of return. If the mud flow rate goes above or drops below the set rate, the system recognizes the change and sends a signal to the readout on the driller's console. If a kick has started, the volume of mud flowing out of the annulus usually increases. The important thing, however, is a change in the mud flow rate. The mud flow indicator can provide the first indication of such a change.

The system should be periodically tested to insure proper operation. Turning off the mud pump can easily do this. When the flow stops coming out of the annulus, the pump is restarted. The indicator should reflect the change in the mud flow rate. In addition, the paddle should be kept clean of any mud accumulation.

Pit Level Indicators

A pit level indicator measures the amount of mud in the tanks (fig. 106) and transfers the information to an indicator on the driller's console (fig. 107). The system consists of several floats in the mud tanks (pits). The floats rise or fall as the level of mud in the tanks changes. This movement registers on a sensor. The sensor sends a signal to a gauge or computer readout on the driller's console. The readout reflects the change in barrels (cubic metres) to provide an easily recognized indication of the severity of the increase or decrease. An automatic alarm is usually incorporated into the system.

Maintenance consists of periodically cleaning the ball floats, checking the paper and ink on the recorder (if one of these old-fashioned devices is still in use), and testing the overall system. As you manually lift each of the floats, the movement should register as a mud level increase on the readout or indicator.

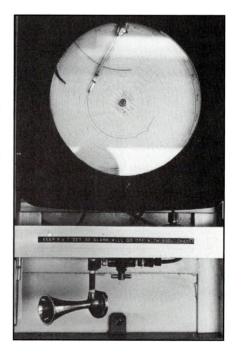

Figure 107.

Mud Volume Measuring Devices

When tripping out pipe, the level of mud in the hole should fall in direct proportion to the volume of pipe pulled out. Since the level of mud decreases, the hydrostatic pressure also decreases. Therefore, mud must be periodically added to the hole to keep it full. Kicks can be hard to detect since the mud level in the well is constantly changing. In addition, mud is not being circulated. Therefore, the mud flow indicator and the pit volume indicator are not very useful.

The primary method of determining if a kick has occurred when tripping is to keep track of how much mud it takes to refill the hole. There are two common ways for the driller to determine how much mud should be pumped back into the hole—mud measuring instruments and trip tanks.

Mud volume can be measured by a series of electronic instruments mounted in the hole fill-up line with a readout device located on the driller's console. Electronic mud measuring devices operate on the principle that the mud pump moves the same amount of mud on every stroke. For instance, say the pump puts out ¼ barrel (40 litres) of mud every stroke (this figure is determined in advance). If it takes 24 strokes to refill the well, then a total of 6 barrels (954 litres) of mud will be needed to refill the well. The driller has the pipe specifications and can calculate just how much mud should be pumped back into the well. If the well takes less mud, then a kick may have started. Taking more mud than calculated indicates possible lost returns.

The instrument often consists of a light that blinks on when the mud pump starts to operate. Another light goes on when the mud starts flowing out of the flow (return) line. This light indicates that the hole is full. The number of pump strokes registers on a separate counter (fig. 108), and, often, a digital readout displays the number of strokes it took to refill the hole the last time. With this information, the driller knows when the mud pump starts, when the hole is full, how many strokes of the pump are needed to fill the hole, and how many strokes were needed to fill the hole previously.

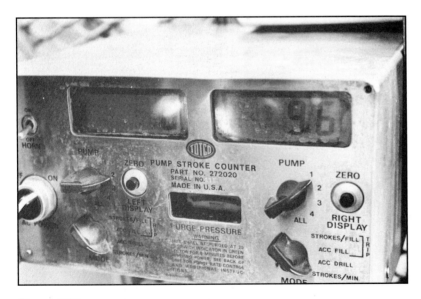

Figure 108.

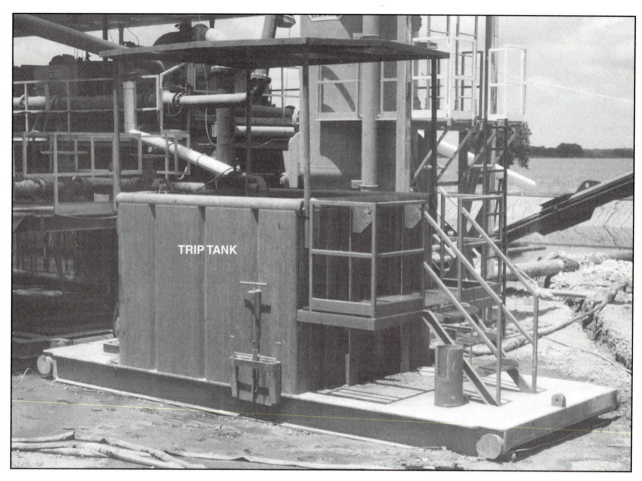

Figure 109.

Maintenance of these instruments consists of periodically checking the flow-line sensors and insuring that the switches and lights are working properly.

The most accurate way of measuring the amount of mud needed to refill the hole is by using a trip tank, a small calibrated holding tank that contains mud (fig. 109). It is usually calibrated in gallons, ¼ barrels, or litres. When the desired number of stands are tripped out, the correct amount of mud from the trip tank to replace the stands is pumped into the well. If the correct amount of mud from the tank fills the hole, (if the hole takes the correct amount of fill-up mud) a kick probably has not occurred. If the hole takes too little mud (it overflows before all the correct amount of mud goes into the hole), then formation fluids may have been swabbed into the hole. If the hole is not full after the correct amount of fill-up mud has been put into the hole, then lost circulation may be occurring.

Gas Detectors

Gas-cut mud is usually first detected by an automatic sensor (fig. 110) that sends a signal to the mud logger. Some type of sensor in or near the return line senses gas in the returning mud and sends a signal to the mud logger's instruments. Other sensors may be located around the mud tanks, in the cellar, or in other confined spaces where gas may accumulate. These sensors warn the crew about any gas accumulations that could result in an explosion or fire.

Gas sensors can be tested with a little lighter fluid or butane fuel spilled on a rag. This small amount of gas should activate the alarm. Any broken lines, dirty sensors, or other visible problems should be repaired immediately.

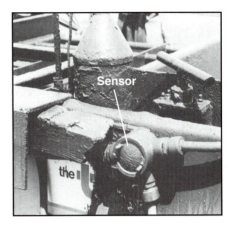

Figure 110.

Degassers

If gas-cut mud is encountered while drilling, the fluid must be channeled through a degasser before it can be recirculated down the well. A degasser uses mechanical means to separate the gas from the mud. One popular type is a vacuum degasser (fig. 111). The gas-mud mixture is pumped into one side of the unit. It then passes over a baffle plate inside the degasser. The thin film of mud on the baffle plate allows the vacuum inside the tank to pull gas out of the fluid. The gas is usually flared. The degassed mud flows out of the degasser and back into the mud pits.

General maintenance of the unit includes checking the oil level and belts, examining the float control arm and three-way valve for movement, and testing the unit for leaks.

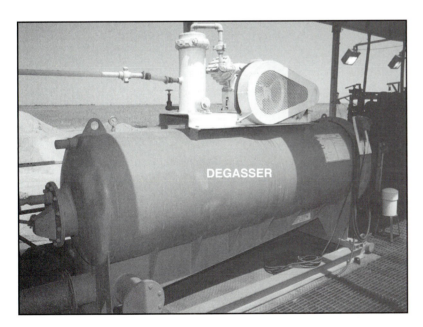

Figure 111.

A

abnormal pressure *n:* formation pressure higher or lower than the normal pressure expected at a given depth. In the Gulf Coast of the U.S., normal pressure increases about 0.465 psi per foot (10.519 kPa per metre) of depth. Thus, normal pressure at 10,000 feet is 4,650 psi or at 1,000 metres normal pressure is 10.519 kPa. Formations with abnormally high pressure must be controlled to prevent a blowout.

accumulator *n:* see *blowout preventer control unit.*

adjustable choke *n:* a special valve that has an adjustable opening. It is usually located in the choke manifold. Usually, an adjustable choke can be controlled from a remote location by means of a choke control panel. The choke's opening can be completely closed, completely opened, or adjusted to any size in between the two extremes. It is used to control the flow out of the annulus while venting a kick and to hold the correct amount of back-pressure on the well to keep bottomhole pressure constant.

annular blowout preventer *n:* a large valve, usually installed above the ram preventers on a blowout preventer stack. It forms a seal in the annular space between the pipe and the wellbore, or, if no pipe is in the well, it can seal the open hole.

B

background gas *n:* a small amount of gas that appears in the returning mud as the hole is being drilled. It is caused by drilling through a formation containing small amounts of gas, which mix with the drilling mud as the bit cuts through the rock.

barite *n:* barium sulfate, a mineral used to increase the weight of the drilling mud. Its specific gravity is 4.2 (i.e., it is 4.2 times heavier than water).

blowout *n:* an uncontrolled flow of gas, oil, or other well fluids into the atmosphere or into an underground formation. A blowout occurs when formation pressure exceeds the pressure applied to it by the column of drilling fluid. A kick warns of an impending blowout.

blowout preventer control unit *n:* a device that stores hydraulic fluid under high pressure and that, when actuated either remotely or by controls on the unit itself, opens or closes the blowout preventers.

blowout preventers *n pl:* equipment installed at the wellhead at the surface level on land rigs and bottoms-supported offshore units and on the seafloor of floating offshore rigs to prevent the escape of pressure either from the annular space between the casing and drill pipe or from an open hole during drilling and completion operations.

blowout preventer stack *n:* a series of large valves (blowout preventers) vertically arranged over the wellbore. The stack usually contains one or two annular preventers and several ram preventers.

bottomhole pressure *n:* the pressure in a well at the bottom of the mud column. When mud is being circulated and the bit is drilling ahead, it is the hydrostatic pressure plus the remaining circulating pressure that is lost to friction in the annulus. When circulation is stopped, it is only the hydrostatic pressure of the mud column.

Glossary

C

circulating pressure *n*: the pressure generated by the mud pumps and exerted on the drill stem by the movement of the drilling fluid created by the friction of the mud against everything it comes in contact with in the well.

concurrent method *n*: a method for killing well pressure in which circulation is commenced immediately and mud weight is brought up in a series of circulations, according to a definite schedule. Also called the circulate-and-weight method.

connection gas *n*: formation gas that bleeds into the wellbore when circulation is halted during a connection.

cuttings *n pl*: the fragments of rock dislodged by the bit and brought to the surface in the drilling mud. Washed and dried samples of the cuttings are analyzed by geologists to obtain information about the formations drilled.

D

degasser *n*: the equipment used to remove unwanted gas from a liquid, especially from drilling fluid.

density *n*: the weight of a substance per unit of volume. For instance, the density of a drilling mud may be 10 pounds per gallon (ppg), 74.8 pounds per cubic foot (pcf) or 1,200 kilograms per cubic metre (kg/m³). Specific gravity or API gravity is also a measure of density.

directional drilling *n*: intentional deviation of a wellbore from the vertical. Although wellbores can be drilled vertically, it is sometimes necessary or advantageous to drill at an angle from the vertical. Controlled directional drilling makes it possible to reach subsurface areas laterally remote from the point where the bit enters the earth.

diverter *n*: a system used to control blowouts encountered at relatively shallow depths and to protect floating rigs during blowouts by directing the flow away from the rig.

driller's BOP control panel *n*: a set of controls usually located near the driller's position on the rig floor that allows the blowout preventers to be opened and closed.

driller's method *n*: a well-killing method involving two complete and separate circulations; the first vents the kick out of the well, and the second circulates heavier mud through the wellbore.

drilling break *n*: a change— sometimes sudden—in the rate of penetration by the drill bit. It sometime indicates that the bit has penetrated a high-pressure zone and thus warns of the possibility of a kick.

drill pipe pressure gauge *n*: an indicator that is mounted on the mud circulating system to measure the amount of pressure in the drill stem.

F

flow test *n*: a test to determine if a kick has occurred. First, the mud pump is shut down, stopping circulation; after a short wait to allow the pump to come to a complete stop (about 15-30 seconds), the mud return line is observed for flow. If the flow of mud continues, then a kick has likely occurred.

formation fracturing *n*: in drilling, the process of the formation splitting or cracking. This is caused when the drilling fluid pressure exceeds formation pressure. If the formation cracks, the drilling fluid can flow out of the wellbore into the formation (lost circulation), which may result in a kick as the hydrostatic pressure decreases.

formation pressure *n*: the force exerted by fluids in a formation. It is usually recorded in the hole at the level of the formation with the well shut in. It is also called reservoir pressure.

friction loss *n*: a reduction in the pressure of a fluid caused by its movement against an enclosed surface (as a pipe, jet nozzle, or wellbore) and within the fluid itself. As the fluid moves through the pipe, friction between the fluid and the pipe wall creates a pressure loss. The faster the fluid moves, the greater the losses are.

G

gas-cut mud *n*: a drilling mud that contains formation gas giving the mud a characteristically fluffy texture. When the gas is not removed from the mud before the mud is returned to the well, the weight or density of the fluid column is reduced, which can result in a kick and possible blowout.

gas detector *n*: a type of sensor that automatically detects gas concentrations in the atmosphere or dissolved in the mud. They are usually located in the return line, around the mud tanks, and in the cellar or other enclosed space. Often an automatic alarm system is incorporated into the sensors.

H

hydrostatic pressure *n*: the force exerted by a body of fluid at rest. The hydrostatic pressure increases directly with the weight and depth of the fluid. In drilling, hydrostatic pressure usually refers to the pressure exerted by the drilling fluid in the wellbore.

I

initial circulating pressure *n*: the pressure put out by the rig's mud pump plus shut-in drill pipe pressure. This is the circulating pressure used when well-killing procedures start. With the driller's method, initial circulating pressure is maintained throughout the entire first circulation that vents the kick.

inside blowout preventer *n*: a valve installed in the drill stem to prevent a blowout inside the drill stem. Flow is thus possible only downward, allowing mud to be pumped in but preventing any flow back up the stem.

K

kelly cock *n*: a valve installed at the upper end of the kelly. Usually, an upper kelly cock and a lower kelly cock are installed above and below the kelly. When a high-pressure backflow begins inside the drill stem, the valve is closed to keep pressure off the swivel and rotary hose.

kick *n*: the entry of enough water, gas, oil, or other formation fluid into the wellbore to create pressure on the surface when the pumps are stopped and the well is completely shut in. It can occur because the pressure exerted by the column of drilling fluid is not great enough to overcome the pressure exerted by the fluids in the formation. It can also occur if too much formation fluid is swabbed into the well during a trip. If prompt action is not taken to control the kick, or kill the well, a blowout can occur.

kill rate *n*: the speed at which the mud pump operates during well-killing procedures. Usually, several kill-rate speeds are chosen in advance of any possible kick, and they are usually much slower than the normal pumping rate, such as ¾, ⅓, ½ normal pumping rate.

kill-rate pressure *n*: the amount of circulating pressure produced with the mud pump operating at the kill rate. This pressure is usually measured on the drill pipe pressure gauge.

kilopascal *n*: an SI unit of measure for pressure. Abbreviated kPa.

L

lost circulation *n*: the loss of quantities of whole mud to a formation, usually in cavernous, fissured, or coarsely permeable beds, evidenced by the complete or partial failure of the mud to return to the surface as it is being circulated in the hole. Lost circulation can lead to a blowout and, in general, reduce the efficiency of the drilling operation. It is also called lost returns.

M

megapascal *n*: an SI unit of measure for pressure. Abbreviated as MPa.

mud *n*: the liquid circulated through the wellbore during rotary drilling and workover operations. In addition to its function of bringing cuttings to the surface, drilling mud cools and lubricates the bit and drill stem, protects against blowouts by holding back subsurface pressures, and deposits a mud cake on the wall of the borehole to prevent loss of fluids to the formation.

mud flow indicator *n*: a device that continually measures and records the volume of mud returning from the annulus and flowing out of the mud return line. The mud should flow at a fairly constant rate. However, if the rate increases or decreases, it may indicate a kick has occurred or lost circulation.

mud-gas separator *n*: a device in which gas is removed from mud when the well is being circulated through a choke because the well has kicked. The gas is vented a safe distance away, and gas-free mud is returned to the pits.

mud return line *n*: a pipe placed between the surface connections at the wellbore and the shale shaker, through which drilling mud flows upon its return to the surface from down the hole; usually called the flow line.

N

normal pressure *n*: formation fluid pressure equivalent, in the U.S. Gulf Coast, to about 0.465 psi per foot (10.519 kPa per metre) of depth from the surface. If the formation pressure is 4,650 at 10,000 feet (10,519 kPa at 1,000 metres), it is considered normal in the Gulf Coast. In other areas, normal pressure may vary somewhat from 0.465 (10.519), but only by a few decimal points.

P

permeable rock *n*: a porous rock formation in which the individual pore spaces are connected, allowing fluids to flow through the formation.

pit-level indicator *n*: a device that continuously monitors the level of drilling mud in the mud tanks (pits). An indicator usually consists of float devices in the mud tanks that sense the mud level and transmit data to a recording and alarm device mounted near the driller's position on the rig floor. If the mud level drops too low or rises too high, the alarm sounds to warn the driller that action may be necessary to shut in the well to control a kick.

porous rock *n*: a rock or rock formation containing small openings or spaces within the rock. The spaces are often filled with fluid (such as water, oil, gas, or all three).

pounds per gallon (ppg) *n*: a measure of the density or weight of drilling fluid.

pounds per square inch (psi) *n*: an English measure of the amount of pressure on an area that is 1-inch square.

pressure *n*: the force that a fluid (liquid or gas) exerts when it is in some way confined within a vessel, pipe, or hole in the ground, such as that exerted against the inner wall of a tank or that exerted on the bottom of the wellbore by drilling mud. Pressure is often expressed in terms of force per unit of area, as pounds per square inch (psi), or kilograms per cubic meter (kg/m^3). In the SI system of measurement, pressure is expressed in kilopascals (kPa) or megapascals (MPa).

pressure gradient *n*: a scale of pressure differences in which there is a uniform variation of pressure from point to point. For example, the pressure gradient of a column of fresh water is about 0.433 psi/foot (9.795 kPa/metre) of vertical elevation. The normal pressure gradient in a well is often expressed as equivalent to the pressure exerted at any given depth by a column of 10 percent salt water extending from that depth to the surface (i.e., 0.465 psi/foot or 10.519 kPa/metre).

R

ram blowout preventer *n*: a blowout preventer that uses rams to seal off pressure inside a hole that either does or does not have pipe in it. It is also called ram preventer. Three types of ram preventers are a pipe ram, a shear ram, and a blind ram. Pipe ram preventers seal around drill pipe in the hole; shear ram preventers cut drill pipe and form a seal; and blind ram preventers seal on open hole (hole with no pipe in it).

remote blowout preventer panel *n*: a set of controls used to open and close the blowout preventers; placed some distance away from the rig so that they can be operated without personnel present on the rig floor.

rotary torque *n*: resistance of the drill string to being rotated.

S

shut in *v*: to close the blowout preventers and the choke on a well sealing the well against a kick.

shut-in casing pressure (SICP) *n*: pressure of the annular fluid on the casing when the well is shut in.

shut-in drill pipe pressure (SIDPP) *n*: the pressure on the drill pipe gauge when the well is shut in and the mud pump is off. The reading represents the difference between the hydrostatic pressure of the drilling fluid and the formation pressure.

sub *n*: a short, threaded piece of pipe used to adapt parts of the drilling string that cannot otherwise be screwed together because of differences in thread size or design. A sub may also perform a special function. Lifting subs are used with drill collars to provide a shoulder to fit the drill pipe elevators. A kelly saver sub is placed between the drill pipe and kelly to prevent excessive thread wear of the kelly and drill pipe threads. A bent sub is used when drilling a directional hole. Sub is a short expression for substitute.

surging *n*: a rapid increase in downhole pressure that occurs when the drill stem is lowered too fast or when the mud pump is rapidly brought up to speed after starting.

swabbing *n*: the phenomenon by which drilling fluid tends to adhere to the drill stem as it is pulled from the hole. Formation fluid can be swabbed into the hole leading to a kick.

T

tripping *n*: the operation of hoisting the drill stem out of and returning it to the wellbore; making a trip.

trip tank *n*: a small mud tank that is calibrated in small divisions, such as gallons, ¼ barrels, or litres, that is used to ascertain the amount of mud that is put into the hole to replace the volume occupied by the pipe removed from the hole. When pipe is pulled out of the hole, a volume of mud equal to that which the drill pipe occupied while in the hole must be placed into the hole to replace the pipe. When pipe goes back in the hole, the pipe displaces a certain amount of mud, and a trip tank again can be used to keep track of this volume.

true vertical depth *n*: the depth of a well measured from the surface straight down to the bottom of the well. The true vertical depth of a well may be quite different from its actual measured depth, because wells are very seldom drilled exactly vertical.

W

wait-and-weight method *n*: a well-killing method in which the well is shut in and the mud weight is raised to the required amount to kill the well. The heavy mud is then circulated into the well while at the same time the kick fluids are circulated out; so called, because one shuts the well in and waits for the mud to be weighted before circulating begins.

well control *n*: the methods and techniques used to prevent a well from blowing out. Such techniques include but are not limited to keeping the borehole completely filled with drilling mud of the proper weight, or density, during all operations, exercising reasonable care when tripping pipe out of the hole to prevent swabbing, and keeping careful track of the amount of mud put into the hole to replace the volume of pipe removed from the hole during a trip.

INTRODUCTION TO WELL CONTROL

Multiple Choice

Pick the *best* answer from the choices and place the letter of that answer in the blank provided. (In some cases, but not always, more than one answer is required.)

1. You are working on a drilling rig and the well is 14,823 feet (4,518.1 metres) deep. The drilling rate recently increased from 4 feet per hour to 6 feet per hour (1.22 metres per hour to 1.83 metres per hour). The mud engineer told you to tell the driller that the chloride content (salt content) of the returning mud has increased. Also, the derrickhand noticed that the cuttings have increased in size. The driller shut off the mud pump, and there is no flow from the mud return line. In the situation described above, a kick probably—
   a. could occur.
   b. could not occur.
   c. has occurred.

2. The warning signs that occurred in question 1 were—
   a. a drilling break.
   b. a change in cutting size.
   c. a change in the mud composition.
   d. all of the above

3. The first warning sign to appear was a—
   a. change in the mud's composition.
   b. change in cutting size.
   c. drilling break.
   d. the driller yelling, "Be careful."

4. This situation was probably caused by—
   a. increasing the drilling speed.
   b. a dull bit.
   c. drilling into a new type of formation.
   d. drilling below 14,000 feet (4,267 metres).

5. The wellbore is 9,870 feet (3,008.4 metres) deep. For the last two hours, gas cut mud has been appearing in the tanks. The cuttings have recently gotten smaller and the volume, or amount, of cuttings falling on the shale shaker has decreased significantly. Suddenly, the alarm that warns of an increase in the return mud flow rate sounds. In this situation, a kick probably—
   a. has occurred.
   b. has not occurred.
   c. could occur.
   d. could not occur.

_____ 6. In the situation in question 5, the first indication that a kick might occur was the—
   a. tank volume alarm.
   b. reduction in the number of cuttings.
   c. gas-cut mud flowing from the well.
   d. lack of an increase in flow from the mud return line.

_____ 7. A good way to absolutely determine whether a kick has occurred is to—
   a. check the mud tank volume.
   b. shut the pump down and check for flow.
   c. close in the well.
   d. none of the above

_____ 8. If the pump is shut down and the well does not flow, it most likely means that a—
   a. kick has occurred.
   b. kick has not occurred.
   c. kick will probably occur.
   d. both a and c

_____ 9. The bit is drilling at 12,837 feet (3,912.7 metres) at a steady 5 feet (1.52 metres) per hour. The cuttings have remained constant in size and amount, and no sign of gas-cut mud exists. The crew began a trip out of the hole about an hour ago. Instructions are to fill the hole after each stand of drill collars is pulled. The hole has taken 6½ barrels (103.4 decalitres) of mud for each stand of drill collars that have been tripped out, which matches each drill collar stand's displacement. With the pump off, the well does not flow. In this case, a kick probably—
   a. has occurred.
   b. has not occurred.
   c. could occur.

_____ 10. In the situation described in question 9, how many kick warning signs are present?
   a. 3
   b. 2
   c. 1
   d. 0

_____ 11. If the well suddenly starts to flow when the pump is off—
   a. a kick could occur.
   b. a kick has occurred.
   c. the stands should be tripped out slower.
   d. none of the above

_____ 12. If the well described in question 9 starts to take 2 barrels (32 decalitres) of mud per tripped drill collar stand—
   a. a kick has probably occurred.
   b. a kick has not occurred.
   c. lighter mud should be used.
   d. the mud pump speed should be increased.

_____ 13. The hole has reached a depth of 10,983 feet (3,347.6 metres), and the crew has been tripping out of the hole for the last hour. While on bottom and drilling just before the trip, the drilling rate increased from 10 feet (3 metres) per hour to 14 feet (4.3 metres) per hour with a slight increase in rotary torque. The mud was not gas cut, nor did any changes appear in the cuttings on the shaker. As the last two stands are pulled from the hole, the hole stays full of mud. In this situation, a kick probably—
   a. has occurred.
   b. has not occurred.
   c. could occur.
   d. could not occur.

_B_____ 14. In question 13, the first indication that a kick could occur was—
    a. flow from the mud return line.
    b. a drilling break.
    c. no increase in cutting size.
    d. an increase in rotary torque.

_C_____ 15. In question 13, you can tell the well has kicked by the—
    a. lack of gas-cut mud.
    b. increase in rotary torque.
    c. hole's not taking the correct amount of mud.
    d. changes in the cutting size.

_C_____ 16. A kick occurs when—
    a. hydrostatic pressure exceeds formation pressure.
    b. drilling fluid flows into the formation.
    c. formation fluids flow into the wellbore.
    d. hydrostatic and circulating pressure are equal.

_A_____ 17. Pressure is usually measured in the U.S. in—
    a. pounds per square inch.
    b. pounds per square foot.
    c. pounds per gallon.
    d. grams per square centimetre.

_C_____ 18. Fluid density refers to a fluid's—
    a. thickness.
    b. depth.
    c. weight.
    d. viscosity.

_b_____ 19. Formation pressure refers to the pressure exerted by—
    a. formation rock.
    b. formation fluid.
    c. both a and b.

_b_____ 20. In a well full of drilling fluid, the hydrostatic pressure at the bottom of the well depends on the well's—
    a. total measured depth.
    b. true vertical depth.
    c. depth and diameter.
    d. rate of penetration.

Matching

Place the letter from the correct definition on the right in the blank at left to properly define each term.

_D_____ 21. psi

_C_____ 22. formation pressure

_G_____ 23. hydrostatic pressure

_b_____ 24. swabbing

_F_____ 25. surging

_A_____ 26. lost circulation

_E_____ 27. formation fracture

a. drilling fluid flowing into the formation

b. caused by tripping out too fast

c. pressure exerted by fluid in a rock

d. measurement of pressure in the U.S.

e. caused by surging

f. momentary increase in hydrostatic pressure

g. pressure exerted by drilling fluid

Comparsion

Compare the two lists of pressure readings, and if you think a kick could occur, check the box under *Yes*, but if you don't think a kick could occur, check the box under *No*. Don't use any other information or considerations except the two pressure readings.

	Yes	No	Formation Pressure	Hydrostatic Pressure
28.	☑	☐	5,756 psi	5,253 psi
29.	☐	☑	7,392 psi	7,645 psi
30.	☑	☐	39,344 kPa	28,298 kPa
31.	☐	☑	3,678 psi	3,987 psi
32.	☑	☐	48,766 kPa	47,475 kPa

Multiple Choice

Pick the *best* answer from the choices and place the letter of that answer in the blank provided. (In some cases, but not always, more than one answer is required.)

___C___ 33. The greatest amount of circulating pressure is lost as drilling mud passes through the—
   a. annulus.
   b. drill stem.
   c. bit nozzles.
   d. return line.

___B___ 34. A drilling break means—
   a. the drill pipe has broken (twisted off).
   b. a change in the drilling rate.
   c. the end of the tour.
   d. the time it takes to make a trip.

___B___ 35. You can usually notice a change in the cutting size at the—
   a. mud pump.
   b. shale shaker.
   c. driller's console.
   d. jet hopper.

___C___ 36. Gas-cut mud is usually observable at the—
   a. mud pump.
   b. driller's console.
   c. mud tanks (pits).
   d. rotary hose.

The hole is at 12,837 feet (3,913 metres). The rate of penetration has been a steady 12 feet (3.5 metres) per hour, the cuttings have remained the same size and amount, and no gas-cut mud has showed up. The crew started out of the hole about 30 minutes ago. The driller knows that each stand of drill collars near the bottom of the string displaces 7 barrels (111.3 decalitres) of mud. The driller has been filling the hole after each stand of collars is pulled. After pulling the first five stands, the hole has taken a total of 35 barrels (556.5 decalitres) of mud. No one has seen any fluid flowing from the well.

___B___ 37. In the above situation, a kick probably—
   a. has occurred.
   b. has not occurred.

_D____ 38. There are _____ warning signs present.

    a. 3

    b. 2

    c. 1

    d. 0

_B____ 39. In the above situation, the crew continues with the trip. After another drill collar stand is pulled, the well takes 5 barrels (80 decalitres) to fill.

    a. A blowout is underway.

    b. Formation fluids have probably been swabbed into the hole.

    c. No need to worry; the trip tank is probably inaccurate.

    d. Surging has forced more mud into the well from the tanks.

You are drilling at a depth of 1,870 metres (6,135 feet). The derrickhand reports to the driller that the cuttings falling onto the shaker have gotten smaller and fewer of them seem to be coming out of the hole. Also, there has been an increase in the rate of penetration. No one has noticed any gain in the mud tanks. All of sudden the return line indicator alarm begins to sound.

_A____ 40. In the above situation, a kick probably—

    a. has occurred.

    b. has not occurred.

    c. could occur.

    d. could not occur.

_B____ 41. A good way to determine whether a kick has occurred is to—

    a. check the mud tank (pit) volume.

    b. shut the pump off and check for flow.

    c. check with the toolpusher.

    d. none of the above

The rig is drilling at 14,823 feet (4,518 metres). The drilling rate has gradually increased from about 4 feet (1.2 metres) per hour to about 6 feet (1.8 metres) per hour. The mud engineer has reported to the driller that the chloride content (salinity) of the mud has increased a small amount. Being a careful person, the driller stops rotating, picks the bit up off bottom, shuts down the pump, and looks for flow from the mud return line. After waiting a few moments, no mud flows out of the return line.

_B____ 42. In the situation described above, a kick probably—

    a. has occurred.

    b. has not occurred.

_A____ 43. Were there any kick warning signs at all?

    a. yes

    b. no

_C____ 44. The situation was probably caused by—

    a. a dull bit.

    b. drilling below 14,000 feet (4,267 metres).

    c. drilling into a new formation.

    d. none of the above

The well is 7,890 feet (2,405 metres) TVD. About half the drill stem has been tripped back into the hole. Mud has flowed from the return line as each stand is lowered into the hole but stopped shortly after the stand was hung in the rotary. As the last few stands were tripped in, the period of no-flow became shorter. As the next stand is being stabbed, you notice that mud flow from the return line has not stopped at all.

_____A_____ 45. In the above situation, a kick probably—
   a. has occurred.
   b. has not occurred.

_____B_____ 46. The first indication that a kick might occur was—
   a. the hole's not taking the right amount of fill-up mud.
   b. shortening periods of no-flow.
   c. a continual flow.
   d. shows of oil in the returning mud.

_____C_____ 47. A good indication that a kick might occur when tripping out of the hole is—
   a. constant flow of mud from the hole.
   b. a tank volume gain.
   c. the hole's not taking the right amount of fill-up mud.
   d. an increase in rotary torque.

In the spaces provided, place a D if the statement refers to the driller's method, place a W if the statement refers to the wait-and-weight method, and place a C if the statement refers to the concurrent method. (Note: some statements may be characteristic of more than one method.)

_____D_____ 48. It has two complete and separate circulations.

_____W_____ 49. SIDPP slowly decreases as the kick is being circulated out of the well.

_____D_____ 50. It exerts the highest pressures on the casing and casing shoe.

__W__C__ 51. Mud weight is increased before the first circulation.

_____D_____ 52. The fewest amount of calculations are required.

_____C_____ 53. The greatest amount of calculations are involved.

_____D_____ 54. SIDPP is kept constant while venting the kick.

_____D_____ 55. The kick is vented before the mud weight is increased.

Multiple Choice

Pick the best answer from the choices and place the letter of that answer in the blank provided. (In some cases, but not always, more than one answer is required.)

_____B_____ 56. After crew members discover a well kick, the first step should be to—
   a. increase the mud weight.
   b. shut in the well.
   c. reduce pump speed.
   d. determine SIDPP.

_____D_____ 57. When circulating with a shut-in well, the drill pipe pressure gauge registers—
   a. hydrostatic pressure in the drill stem.
   b. circulating pressure.
   c. the difference between hydrostatic and formation pressures.
   d. both b and c.

102

_B_ 58. The greatest circulating pressure loss usually occurs—
   a. in the drill stem.
   b. at the bit nozzles.
   c. in the annulus.
   d. at the return line.

_A_ 59. If the well is shut in on a gas kick—
   a. the kick continues to rise up the annulus.
   b. the kick remains at approximately the same pressure.
   c. SICP registers about the same pressure as SIDPP.
   d. SICP registers lower than SIDPP.

_A_ 60. If a kick occurs and the well is not shut in—
   a. a blowout is likely to occur.
   b. it is okay to continue normal operations.
   c. the mud-gas separator can handle the kick.
   d. none of the above

_D_ 61. The well is shut in by using the—
   a. mud-gas separator.
   b. choke manifold.
   c. diverter system.
   d. BOPs.

_A_ 62. After the well is shut in—
   a. there is a limited amount of time to vent the kick.
   b. the kick is permanently stabilized.
   c. a wild-well control specialist is usually brought in.
   d. the hole is abandoned.

_B_ 63. After a well is shut in, 500 psi (3,448 kPa) registers on the casing pressure gauge, which means—
   a. normal drilling operations can continue.
   b. a kick has occurred.
   c. the casing is too weak for the well.
   d. a remedial cementing job is needed.

_D_ 64. If the hydrostatic pressure developed by the mud at the bottom of the hole is 1,400 psi (9,653 kPa) and SIDPP is 400 psi (2,758 kPa), the new formation pressure is—
   a. 400 psi (2,758 kPa).
   b. 1,000 psi (6,895 kPa).
   c. 1,400 psi (9,653 kPa).
   d. 1,800 psi (12,411 kPa).

_A_ 65. Kill-rate pressure is usually determined _____ the kick occurs.
   a. before
   b. when
   c. after

_C_ 66. Initial circulating pressure (ICP) is determined by adding the—
   a. kill-rate pressure.
   b. SIDPP.
   c. both a and b

_B_____ 67. In the wait-and-weight method, as new, heavier mud is being circulated down the drill stem, pressure on the drill pipe pressure gauge—
- a. slowly increases.
- b. slowly decreases.
- c. stays the same.
- d. none of the above

_C_____ 68. In the driller's method, once the kick is circulated out of the well and the well is shut in, the next step is to—
- a. open the BOPs.
- b. recirculate the old mud.
- c. circulate new, heavier mud.
- d. abandon the well.

_D_____ 69. During a well kill, bottomhole pressure is kept constant by adjusting the—
- a. pump speed.
- b. level of mud in the tanks constant.
- c. BOPs.
- d. size of the choke's opening.

_A_____ 70. SICP is usually higher than SIDPP because most kicks —
- a. contain gas or are all gas.
- b. are salt water.
- c. shrink in size as they rise up the hole.
- d. none of the above

Answers

1. a
2. d
3. c
4. c
5. a
6. c
7. b, c
8. b
9. b
10. d
11. b
12. a
13. a
14. b
15. c
16. c
17. a
18. c
19. b
20. b
21. d
22. c
23. g
24. b
25. f
26. a
27. e
28. yes
29. no
30. yes
31. no
32. yes
33. c
34. b
35. b

36. c
37. b
38. d
39. b
40. a
41. b
42. b
43. a
44. c
45. a
46. b
47. c
48. D
49. W
50. D
51. W, C
52. D
53. C
54. D
55. D
56. b
57. d
58. b
59. a
60. a
61. d
62. a
63. b
64. d
65. a
66. c
67. b
68. c
69. d
70. a